When Food is Your Frenemy

WHEN FOOD IS YOUR FRENEMY

From Obesity to Restored Health

JACOB F. BUSTOS

NEW YORK

LONDON • NASHVILLE • MELBOURNE • VANCOUVER

WHEN FOOD IS YOUR FRENEMY

From Obesity to Restored Health

Published in New York, New York, by Morgan James Publishing. Morgan James is a trademark of Morgan James, LLC. www.MorganJamesPublishing.com

ISBN 9781642793376 paperback
ISBN 9781642793383 eBook
Library of Congress Control Number: 2018913137

Cover Design by:
Rachel Lopez
www.r2cdesign.com

Interior Design by:
Chris Treccani
www.3dogcreative.net

Editorial Assistance by:
Mike Yorkey
www.mikeyorkey.com

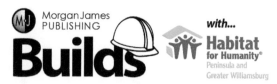

Morgan James is a proud partner of Habitat for Humanity Peninsula and Greater Williamsburg. Partners in building since 2006.

Get involved today! Visit
MorganJamesPublishing.com/giving-back

TABLE OF CONTENTS

A Medical Disclaimer

The purpose of this book is to educate readers. No individual should use the information in this book for self-diagnosis, treatment, or justification in accepting or declining any medical therapy for any health problems or diseases. No individual is discouraged from seeking professional medical advice and treatment, and this book is not supplying medical advice. Any application of the information herein is at the reader's own discretion and risk. Therefore, any individual with a specific health problem or who is taking medications must first seek advice from his personal physician or health-care provider before starting a weight-loss program.

In view of the complex, individual nature of health and fitness problems, this book, and the ideas, programs, procedures, and suggestions herein are not intended to replace the advice of trained medical professionals. All matters regarding one's health require medical supervision. A physician should be consulted prior to adopting any ideas or programs described in this book. The author disclaims any liability arising directly or indirectly from the use of this book.

A Note to the Reader
FROM JACOB BUSTOS

Life change in motion is a concept based on the idea that several paths exist for a person to establish and maintain a healthy relationship with food through the use of portion control. This concept is derived from and inspired by my life experiences as well as my journey from the brink of death to a newly transformed and restored healthy state of life.

Please allow me to introduce myself. I'm Jacob Bustos, a chef and restaurant executive for nearly twenty-five years. I have been in the food industry since my early teenage years, and as I built a successful and rewarding career, serving food to others became my nature.

By the time I reached my early thirties, I had everything going for me, or so it seemed. In hindsight, though, I was in bad shape—physically, mentally, and emotionally. I had always struggled with my weight, but at this point in my life, my weight was spiraling out of control. I was diagnosed with high blood pressure, high cholesterol, diabetes, and a fatty liver, and I needed to do something about my poor health. I tried a zillion diets and promised myself that I would exercise, but I never had much success staying on any program. As my physical health deteriorated, I found myself struggling with severe self-image issues. Being in an industry of high visibility with the public, I felt like I faced daily judgment based on my weight and appearance.

During this time of mental and emotional upheaval, I had a couple of major epiphanies that jolted me to make a change. I came to a realization that the food I loved was my enemy. I was not happy with what I had allowed myself to become.

It was time to set a *life change in motion*, and I committed myself to reducing my weight and restoring my health. First, I recognized that if I was to succeed in my journey to restored health, then I needed to prepare myself mentally for what was to come. After all, one's state of mind is a key factor in achieving goals. I focused my mind on looking forward to a new version of myself, staying positive, and keeping my faith.

Next, after consultations with my doctor and thoroughly researching possible paths forward, I decided to undergo bariatric surgery to initiate my life change in motion. This path, while not for everyone, was what I felt was in my best interest. I pushed through the after effects of the surgery and took my recovery one day at a time. During this process, I learned so much about who I am and what it truly means to love oneself.

I stand now restored in health, mind, and soul. Looking back at my journey, I'm in awe of what I endured and overcame. Submitting to bariatric surgery was no easy feat, and the experiences and near-death instances ignited a further passion and deeper purpose in my life.

Now that I am on the other side of recovery, I have set a plan in motion to tell others about the benefits of my experience and my newfound knowledge. I created the Portion Your Plate program, a concept based on the idea that one can see results by establishing a friendly and healthy relationship with food through using portion control. Within the pages of *When Food Is Your Frenemy* and on my website, PortionYourPlate.com or JacobBustos.com, I promote healthy habits and great-tasting meals through my recipes, cooking demos, podcasts, and videos.

I've set out to use my experiences and my passion for food as a means to encourage others. People face many life challenges, and being overweight with self-image issues is one of the largest areas. To help you get to know me, I will begin by sharing my story, which will give you context and understanding of the journey I've been on.

If I can make a difference in the life of one individual or one child, it makes the journey I've been on all worth it. Ultimately, the choice to make a change rests with you, but I hope that my story will inspire you. From my experience, I pray that you will overcome and survive whatever challenges you may be facing.

Thanks for reading my book. Most importantly, thanks for caring about your future and the state of your health!

1

We All Have a Story

Everyone walking through this world has his or her own story that's a mixture of successes and failures.

I have one as well. The reason I'm sharing my journey is because I feel there is great significance in my story. By sharing my experiences, I believe I can help you through the challenges you're likely facing. Or maybe, just maybe, I can prevent you from making the same mistakes I made. Either way, my goal is to help as many as I can by offering my insights.

It's often said that hindsight is 20/20, and that could not be more of an understatement for me. If only I knew better at an early point in my life. The scars I have would be erased, or at least minimized.

Now when I speak of scars, I mean the literal scars in my abdomen as well as scars not visible to the eye or felt by touch. I'm talking about internal emotional and mental scars. I can best explain going back to beginning.

I come from a small town in New Mexico—Las Vegas, New Mexico, to be exact. Yes, there is a Las Vegas, New Mexico. There aren't any flashy lights or casinos like in the real Las Vegas, but we are from the old Southwest where Billy the Kid came through. We take pride in our families, and we are tight-knit people. Truth be told, it's not uncommon that we know and gather often with family members as far down the line as fourth cousins. It's always food that brings us together.

My parents, who are originally from Las Vegas, raised me and my two siblings in a humble home. I'm lucky enough to have known at least one great-grandparent, and my immediate grandparents from both sides were an active part of my daily life.

I spent many days with my maternal grandparents. I can still remember the days of going to Grandma's house and smelling the fresh flour tortillas she made with her hands. My paternal grandmother always had New Mexico Chile on the stove and fresh apple turnovers on the table, which are still the best I've ever had. My older brother, Anthony, is and always has been my best friend, and my older sister, Jeannette, still remains in New Mexico holding down the family roots.

As a child, I was always self-confident. I did, however, know that I was "chubby" or as my mother would say "husky." I enjoyed being in a leadership role, and my parents still today enjoy telling everyone how I showed up to third grade in a button-down shirt and tie after I was voted class president. You see, I sought a leadership role because of my self-confidence.

As I got into middle school, and the transformation from little boy to pre-teen commenced, I began to develop self-image issues. I wasn't athletic and hated gym class because I was a bit heavier than the other guys. To be honest, kids can be mean and hateful when someone is different than they are.

Struggling to do the same things as other kids my age and being teased for not measuring up really affected the way I thought about myself.

After surviving several turbulent years in middle school, I continued on into high school. With each year, more freedom and more responsibility arose. I decided I wanted what almost every teenager in high school wanted. Yes, a car!

Now, there is another thing you should know about me. When I set my mind to something, there is no stopping me from achieving that goal. My mother would also call me "very determined."

When I asked my parents for a car, the answer I received was, "Sure, as long as you can pay for it." So guess what? I set my mind to figuring out the best way to pay for a car, which obviously meant it was time to get a job. My mother knew the owner of the local McDonald's restaurant. She suggested that I go apply. Actually, she demanded that I go talk to him if I was still determined to get myself a car.

Hence, I applied for my first job at the local McDonald's restaurant. A few days later, I received a call from the hiring manager, and we scheduled an interview. I showed up, walked in the door, got cold feet, left, and went back home. The owner—an acquaintance of my mother— called her and said, "Where is Jacob? He was supposed to interview with us today." My mom sent me right back to the restaurant, and after a perfunctory interview, I was hired. Thus, my career in the restaurant industry was born that day.

Getting a Start

Now, not everyone figures out early in his or her life what he or she wants to be or do for a living, but my goals ever since I can remember were to be a general manager of a restaurant or a hotel.

Remember earlier I said that I come from a close, tight-knit family? Well, one influence in my life was my Aunt Anna. In fact, she enjoyed telling everyone her name was Elizabeth Taylor because her legal married name was Elizabeth Anna Taylor. She got a kick out of that! She was married to my uncle Charles Taylor, and he was the general manager of the local newspaper, the *Las Vegas Daily Optic*. They had a great life and were truly happy. They seemed to have it all—a nice house, nice cars, and nice things. So I wanted to be like my uncle—a general manager.

Looking back at my first job at McDonald's, it was probably not the best job for a teenager who struggled with weight and self-image issues. To top it off, I loved food and I loved to eat. I mean, I loved to eat a lot! And being around food was great, which is why I loved my job and was everything I was looking for—plus it paid for my car, which represented freedom. As my food career began, I loved my job. Working was just what I had hoped for. I did, by the way, get a new car, so it was fitting that I had a good, steady job to pay for the shiny wheels.

I took my newfound responsibilities serving food to the public seriously. I worked hard and learned as much as I could. I showed up for each scheduled shift and outperformed everyone. You see, I had never believed in being mediocre. That's not how I was raised. In fact, I often tell others, "Do it all, or don't do anything."

I also say, "If you don't get things done, then someone else will eat your lunch." Metaphorically speaking, of course. Truth be told, I have always been someone who is aggressive in my goals and who takes pride in giving more than 100 percent effort in every task I undertake. I excelled in my job so much that I was made a shift manager at sixteen years old. I think my boss was crazy to turn over the keys to a million-dollar business to a sixteen-year-old kid, but truth be told, I was more responsible than some of the thirty-year-olds.

When given the chance to be a weekend shift manager, I took it. By the time I turned seventeen, I was asked if I would consider becoming an assistant manager. I was excited and nervous about saying yes. My parents told me that I should think about this decision as it could interfere with attending college.

I thought about the offer and decided that if I really wanted to become a general manager someday, then this was my opportunity to climb one more step toward that goal. I said yes and figured I would worry about its effect on college later. After a month or so on the job, I was told that I excelled at the assistant manager position.

Not only was I a high achiever in my workplace, but I was also a high achiever in school. I had great grades and a high cumulative grade-point average. I was a motivated student and took a lot of core classes my sophomore and junior years, so by my senior year, I only needed to finish two classes to meet graduation requirements.

So, what did this mean? You might have figured out by now that I took every chance to earn as much money as I could. Since my senior schedule allowed me to work as many hours as possible, this allowed me to build up a nice savings account for college.

Truth be told, I let everyone believe my plan was to go to college, but in the back of my mind, I really felt that staying in the restaurant business and making it my career was the best fit for me. First of all, McDonald's training was great. I had been taking management development classes through the McDonald's system. At the time, I had to go to Denver, Colorado, to take one such class, which I did during spring break of my senior year of high school.

Two weeks before my graduation day, I was offered the position of general manager. As chance would have it, the general manager at the time was going to be out of work for months due to a medical issue. I couldn't believe how this worked out so well—as if God has been taking care of me since the very beginning! How could this all have worked out so well? It's as if it was all meant to be. Everything fell into place naturally. I accepted the position of general manager—which meant a nice raise—and graduated from high school in May 1996.

As I continued working as a general manager during the second half of 1996, I began to feel that my future working for a single-store owner/operator of a McDonald's restaurant was limited and would cap my growth potential. I decided that I needed to work in a bigger market with a bigger franchisee, but that meant a move to a bigger city.

Rather than move from Las Vegas, however, I took another job with a different restaurant company at the end of 1996. I hated that job, the way I was treated, and the product we put out. I had already worked for what many felt was the best restaurant concept in the world, which is another reason why the new job was not matching up to my expectations.

One day, a woman walked into our restaurant. I recognized her. She was McDonald's corporate representative who would grade my old store when I was working there.

"Jacob, what are you doing here?" she asked.

I couldn't think of a snappy reply, so I said, "I'm working."

"Can you take a break and have a chat?"

"Sure."

We took a booth, and she told me how talented I was and that I belonged back at McDonald's. "We have an opportunity for you in Albuquerque," she said.

Albuquerque? Hey, why not? It wasn't like I was enjoying where I was.

I moved to Albuquerque and joined PTS Inc., a franchisee of McDonald's. The owner had just purchased a store located off Central Avenue and Rio Grande from a failing franchisee. He wanted me to train new employees in "McDonald's way."

The owner and his Director of Operations decided to send me to their new store, which I quickly learned was in a bad neighborhood with bad employees and a sketchy clientele.

Still, I took on this challenge head-on and persevered. Though it was a team effort, the store became so successful that it was rated AAA by McDonald's. My success was noticed and my talents as a trainer were recognized. From there, the owner had me train over half of the management teams in all his stores—he owned 15—in the Albuquerque area. As I continued to perform well, he offered me the training manager position for the entire Albuquerque market.

Weight Issues Crop Up

Let me pause for a minute and remind you that one of this book's purposes is to share my experiences with respect to the health and weight problems I endured over the majority of my life. Getting to know me and my story will be a significant part of why I feel so strongly about sharing my *life change in motion* concept to help others like you make a change for the better. So while you are reading my story, keep in mind that although everything seems to be going right for me, my weight was continuing to be a problem as it fluctuated up and down. I struggled with self-image issues that weakened my self-confidence. Because my mind was preoccupied with my career, I was neglecting a huge part of myself—my body!

Now, back to my story . . .

In 2002, after more than five years in Albuquerque, the owner I worked for was offered a job as senior vice president of McDonald's for all of the USA, meaning that he and his family had to move to the corporate headquarters in Chicago. He then sold his franchises to the McDonald's corporation, which turned me into a corporate McDonald's employee. During this time, my weight did not fluctuate with up and down movements. Instead, it only went straight up!

When Enough Was Enough

As I approached thirty years old, I was weighing in at two hundred and fifty pounds. Not good for me, I know.

I was visiting my doctor regularly, and he would tell me over and over that I needed to lose the extra weight. Otherwise, he said, I would die of a heart attack or be diagnosed with diabetes, which ran rampant in my father's side of the family. My blood work results were not good, and for the next four years continued to deteriorate. At that point, I was thirty-four and still single, but I wasn't much of a catch. I weighed 320 pounds and felt worse than ever. The only thing that I felt I had going for me was that I was good at my job—training employees for Panera. But even then, I felt there were times when I was viewed poorly by others for being so overweight.

I had heard about bariatric surgery and asked my doctor what he thought about the procedure. He told me that I needed to lose weight the traditional way—performing lots of exercise and eating little food.

Hey, Doc! I work in the restaurant business. Food is my life. I like to cook, and I'm also a chef!

I decided to find a doctor who would understand me better. I found an amazing doctor at Kaiser Permamente who told me that I needed to lose ten pounds. Do that, and I would be considered a candidate for a bariatric procedure.

That seemed doable. I lost ten pounds and made it through the psychological evaluations. In the spring of 2012, I went under the knife. My surgeon did a fantastic job, and even though I was in pain for a while, I knew the outcome would be great.

Over time, I lost 160 pounds, which was amazing. Even though I felt I was at my ideal weight—and life was good—I still felt troubled with self-image issues because of the excess skin left behind from my drastic weight loss. In the fall of 2015, I arranged for another surgery to have the excess skin removed.

In the weeks leading up to the surgery, a strange feeling came over me. Something was telling me that I needed to be prepared for whatever may happen, so at this point, I made my will and included written plans for my funeral services, just in case. My brother, Anthony, having a strong feeling that he should be with me, flew in from Arizona for the procedure, which wasn't like him.

I was wheeled into the operation bay at 6 a.m. I was told that the skin removal procedure would take four hours. After recovery, I would be released to go home in the early afternoon.

Things did not work out that way. At five p.m., I was still in the recovery room and having a tough time coming out of anesthesia.

Nonetheless, I was released and told I could go home. Man, I was woozy. Anthony and my mom, who had also come out from Albuquerque, practically carried me to my living room couch because I couldn't make it to my bedroom on the second floor. I had been told to get into in a fetal position and stay that way for the next two weeks.

I felt so out of it. I tried to sleep in my pain, but I couldn't get comfortable. At nine o'clock, I felt the right side of my abdomen. It felt wet.

"Anthony, can you check this out?"

My brother gingerly touched me. "Dude, you're bleeding." I had been told that I could expect some degree of bleeding, so I figured this was what the doctor was talking about.

An hour later, I called my brother over again. This time, my bandages were soaked in blood. A call was put into my doctor, who told my brother to get me to the emergency room immediately. Even though Anthony wrapped a bath towel over my bandages, I could feel the blood pouring out.

We got in the car with Anthony behind the wheel since I was obviously in no shape to drive. Mom looked awfully worried from the back seat. I can barely remember each moment, but I do remember praying that God would spare my life but that His will be done. I was in dire straights.

When we arrived at the emergency room, I walked in with Anthony's and Mom's help. I was immediately taken to an examination room and placed on a bed. I laid down in a fetal position and was going in and out of consciousness.

My surgeon had rushed to the hospital to see me. "Hang in there," he said as he barked directions to other doctors and nurses. From the nervousness in their voices, I could tell I was in trouble. I was losing so much blood. I heard my doctor calling for a transfusion—and make it snappy.

In that moment, I felt an overwhelming peace come over me. It helped that I could hear Anthony praying for me. In fact, I could hear him praying, but I could not see him. I was in a place of love and peace. I was in the presence of the Lord!

I saw my grandmother who had died a few years before. I saw my Aunt Anna, who had also passed on. I saw a few others I recognized but no one would speak to me. I was watching the doctors and nurses around me, and I could see my mother agonizing over my departure from earth.

Time did not exist, and I was at peace. The rest of that experience is very personal to me, and I choose not to share more at this time, but I will say that as I was in the Lord's presence, He made very clear to me that my job on earth was to feed His people. That made sense to me since I had always been in the food business.

Food is love, it is family, and it is joy. I have learned that we need food to live, but never to overfill. I have learned that Christ walked this earth and asked only to be remembered by a piece of bread and wine. I have learned that it's not important how much money you have, what kind of car you drive, or how big your house is. What matters is what you do with the gifts you've been given.

You see, *nothing* belongs to us. We are allowed to have things, but the focus on material items is not where our attention should be. We will always be blessed with "things" as long as we share with the less fortunate and help those in need.

I survived my surgery, for which I'm thankful because following my recovery, I knew what my purpose and focus should be, which is to share my story with you, in hopes that my experience will resonate with you, touch your heart, and drive you to set your own life change in motion, especially if you're at a pivotal point in your life where something needs to change.

2

My Bariatric Journey

Now you know a little bit more about me, where I come from, and my struggles with weight, self-image, and self-confidence.

You know that I've shared some of my most significant and personal events. I've walked you through my life from childhood to my mid-thirties and described the significant role that food and weight played in my life. You know about my decision to have bariatric surgery, the result of that surgery being significant weight loss, and the decision to undergo surgery for excess skin removal. You also know that I survived it all, as trying as everything was.

In everything we do, we take the good with the bad and hope and pray that in the long run, the good outweighs the bad. I'm here to tell you this has definitely been the case for me. Even with all the "bad," however, I still would make the same decisions that initiated my bariatric journey because the procedure yielded so much positivity for my life.

Since my operation, it's become my mission to tell others and encourage them to change their lives for the better. That's why I feel it's important, at this time, to share my bariatric journey in greater detail so that you can decide whether this route to weight loss can work for you.

It's not my place to tell you which choice to make. That decision will be different for every individual, based upon your life and family situation. Bariatric surgery does require you to take many things into consideration before committing one way or the other.

As you read further, you'll realize the decision to submit to such an invasive surgery cannot be made lightly. I'm hoping my experience will help you to gain a better understanding of the bariatric process and the requirements associated with the procedure. But first, let's backtrack a bit to the point where my bariatric journey began.

How I Got Started

When I was in my mid-thirties, I was BROKEN! What kept me going was knowing that I was still young with a lot of life ahead of me. I had to act and try something I hadn't before—or face a shortened mortality.

Once I spoke to my doctor about bariatric surgery, and he agreed to get the process started, I underwent a complete battery of blood testing to see what the true state of my health was. I knew I was in bad shape, but the numbers really confirmed how poor my health really was.

First of all, I weighed 320 pounds, considered morbidly obese because I was more than 100 pounds overweight. If you are not at least 100 pounds overweight, most doctors will not consider you a good candidate for bariatric surgery unless there are other health risks such as diabetes. I met that criteria as well since my blood work results showed that I had conditions like type 2 diabetes and high cholesterol. The good news was that the prognosis of the surgery and undergoing the regimen that followed meant that these conditions could be resolved.

As part of the screening process, I was sent for a mental health evaluation. Believe it or not, anyone considering gastric bypass, a sleeve gastrectomy, or even the adjustable lap band procedure will likely be required to go through a complete mental health screening.

It's important to understand that you have to be in a good mental state and ready to make a change. This will be crucial to your success with weight loss via the bariatric process. While anyone can say he or she is ready, a mental health screening will ensure that you can mentally handle the changes you have to make to get healthy. If you do not prepare mentally to change, your old lifestyle habits will come right back.

You will have to exercise mind over matter. In a strange way, your body will transform, but it cannot be done without the initial transformation of your mind and thought processes. There is no shortcut to this step because mindset matters. This is Phase 1 of the *life change in motion* concept that I'm introducing, which I will discuss in greater detail in Chapter 4.

A second point is that many people who go through gastric bypass surgery do not keep the weight off. You might be surprised to learn this, but any bariatric procedure is only just a tool.

In order to be successful, there must be commitment and discipline. There will be things you will have to do that will not be easy by any means. Nevertheless you must stick with the program and see things through until the end.

Before surgery, I had to go to classes for thirteen weeks. Many people don't commit to attending class and doing the homework, meaning they won't get approved for bariatric surgery. These classes are important to the success of your weight loss because of what you learn about nutrition and eating certain foods *after* your procedure, as well as the way your body will work. For instance, following bariatric surgery, your body will not absorb nutrients normally anymore. This is why a vitamin regimen is critical to the success of your health transformation.

Third, your health transformation does not end once the surgery is complete and you walk out the hospital; it's only the beginning. In fact, that's when the hard work begins and commitment and discipline are put into action. If you decide to pursue the weight-loss route rather than undergoing a surgical procedure, however, this is where the transformation process can apply to you in terms of the food restrictions and portion limits you should adhere to.

If you cannot commit to making these type of changes, you should not consider any bariatric procedure. As a small example, more than half of people who were in my bariatric classes were unwilling to give up alcoholic beverages. In turn, the nurses and doctors told them that they would not make good candidates for the surgery.

So how badly do you want to lose weight and get healthy? Are you willing to give up drinking alcohol to make that happen?

You see, you will have to give something to get something better in return. Nothing in this life comes without hard work, commitment, dedication, and discipline. I can assure you, though, that the satisfaction you'll feel after seeing what you've accomplished with your weight loss and getting your health back on track will be well worth it.

Getting into a Routine

My post-surgery daily routine goes something like this, but keep in mind that your new routine will be similar but not exact to mine.

Each day, I wake up at 5 a.m. and eat a protein bar or drink a protein shake. For our bodies—whether you have had this procedure or not—one thing is for sure: breakfast is the most important meal of the day.

Think of your body as a fireplace. When you go to sleep, your mind relaxes, as does your body. When you wake up in the morning, you need to stoke the embers of a dying fire. In other words, it's imperative to kick-start your metabolism early in the day. For this reason, you should take in some sort of protein within thirty minutes of waking up.

It's also important to eat a snack mid-morning. Think of it as putting another log in the fireplace. Just like in preschool and the elementary school years, snacks are important. Snack time is good for the body and mind and is something that schools—even into high school—should encourage.

A sensible lunch is also important. Eating a healthy balanced meal during the noon hour will keep your metabolic rate going into the afternoon.

It's also important to keep track of your food intake. Counting calories ensures that you eat balanced meals and keeps you accountable. An afternoon snack—like a small portion of yogurt, nuts, and fresh berries—will give you energy through your afternoon.

I've found dinner to be the trickiest meal. I know that everyone's busy finishing up work and trying to get home while fighting traffic, meaning that some people don't eat until late in the evening—say after 8 p.m. But you want to eat dinner early enough to keep your "fireplace" going but not so late that the flame stays lit late into the night and affects your sleep time. Small dinners in the early evening are a smart way to ensure a restful night of sleep.

Speaking of sleep, this is something that we all need more of. Eight hours of sleep is great if you can get it, which is why I'm often in bed by nine o'clock. Your body resets when you sleep, so if you eat right throughout the day, your body will continue to burn calories at a good rate even while you are sleeping.

Stay away from fast food. I know . . . I worked at McDonald's for many years, but that was before I knew that fast foods were full of sodium and sugars. In fact, anytime you eat a lot of processed foods and restaurant-prepared meals, you're sure to consume the wrong ingredients.

Instead, eat clean. What does that mean? It means eating foods that are free of antibiotics, sugars, artificial colors, and preservatives and are not genetically modified. When you shop the food aisles, stay away from foods that have already been "conveniently" packed for you. Whenever foods are pre-packaged for convenience, it means they likely have been made with preservatives to keep from rotting or spoiling.

Foods that spoil and rot are good foods. Let me explain. If you buy a piece of fresh fruit and set it on your kitchen counter, it will rot or spoil in a few days. That means it was fresh, so you have to eat that fruit within a good time frame. If you buy bread that gets moldy after a few days, that was actually a sign of its freshness. This may not make sense, but when foods have been loaded with chemical preservatives to give it a longer "shelf life," they may last a long time, but they certainly are not the healthiest for you. Fresh, healthy foods should do what food normally does—spoil and rot. Hence *fresh foods* equal *healthy foods*.

Now remember, eating this way may be harder and more of a hassle—since you'll have to shop for fresh foods more often—but the results will be positive. Not only will developing a routine of consuming smaller portions of healthy foods and good quality sleep help you feel better, but you will also see a stark difference in your energy level. This will bring you closer to restored health, a clearer mind, and a happy heart.

The Struggle Is Real

While my journey is unique, I recognize that aspects of my health odyssey are common to many people. I realize that a good number of people are successful in losing weight and/or maintaining a healthy weight. But as the current obesity statistics tell us, struggles with trying to eat healthy and being overweight are real for many people.

I believe the underlying issues dealing with healthy eating and having a healthy weight dwell much deeper inside oneself. When you think of self-image, what's the first thing that comes to your mind? Most likely your initial thoughts center on appearance—how you look to others. The *Cambridge University Press Dictionary* defines self-image as "your opinion of yourself, especially how you appear to other people."

Self-image actually encompasses several more ideas about yourself. This means anything that affects how you view yourself shapes your self-image. In addition, events in your life will likely also affect your self-image. As was the case in my life, weight was a serious negative contributor to my self-image while also impacting my level of self-confidence and self-worth.

One thing I've come to realize is that while I felt totally alone in my situation, that couldn't have been farther from the truth. You see, I now understand something astounding. Everyone, and I do mean every single person, no matter how perfect they may be with respect to appearance, will find a flaw in themselves that will affect their self-image. You see, each of us is his or her own worst critic.

To be fair, we have all been programmed by behaviors we see through media and entertainment channels. We've been programmed to think that we have to strive for some unattainable "image of perfection," yet we all too often fall short of that goal. There's a reason for that—it's unattainable. We look at "perfect" people in movies, TV shows, glamour magazines, or online in social media, but they are not really "perfect" because nearly all the photos you see of them have been "touched up" by professionals paid to make them look their best.

In addition, when you understand that celebrities have access to professional trainers, expensive organic foods, professional chefs who prepare healthy meals, and cosmetic surgery to make them look their best, then you will have the right perspective.

Now you can set your expectations for yourself that are more real . . . and after all, you and I live in the real world!

You can achieve your personal goals and eat healthy even if you don't have the same savings account that the rich and famous do. You can exercise without breaking the bank. If you can't afford a pricey gym, go for a long walk around your neighborhood. Just think: you can meet new people while you're doing so. You can go to the local high school track field and walk or run. Give yourself extra time before work to take the stairs instead of using the elevator. Park further away at the stores and walk just a little bit further to get to the entrance.

These are some of the small tricks to getting in better shape, and I'm sure you have some of your favorite ways of getting some exercise. You'll also need one more crucial concept: You will need to be committed to making this life change. You have to change your mindset and focus on attainable results you can achieve and leave behind the illusion of "perfection" from the big screen.

This is what I was finally able to understand and apply to my life. What a difference that has made, and I want you to make a huge change in your health as well.

If you're still on the fence, think about this for a minute. You live in the wealthiest country in the world. You have access to the best foods and healthcare. You have access to just about anything you may need. Just walk into any store, and you can readily pick up whatever you want and afford to pay for it. In fact, you live in an age where you make a few clicks online and have anything in a matter of hours delivered to your doorstep. So why not use the resources at your fingertips to commit to a life change that will lead you to a happier and healthier restored state of life?

There are no excuses.
The time is now.
Get ready.
Get motivated and set your *life change in motion.*

Next Steps

When I started my life change in motion, I put myself in a position to conquer and overcome the challenges I faced. My life change in motion is based on my personal experiences, and in order for you to clearly understand it, it was important for me to detail background information on my life, my journey with food, my weight, and my self-image issues.

The life change in motion that I've undergone is still unfolding and dynamically changing, but I know I'm heading down the right path. I'm now choosing food as my friend, not my enemy.

Now is the time for me to give you the keys to set your life change in motion. This concept is not a diet plan. This is a lifestyle that is made simple for post-bariatric people, but it's also a guide for people who may not be going through the bariatric process but want to maintain good eating habits so that they can lose weight and get healthier.

Looking ahead, I will present to you gourmet foods made simple, healthy, and focused on portion control. I will bring you a lifestyle enhanced by my personal experience with weight loss and self-image issues. These next chapters focus on the individual phases of my *life change in motion* concept that also incorporate my Portion Your Plate concept, which is essentially eating healthy-portioned meals.

In addition, at the end of my book, you'll find a chapter of my best and healthy recipes to get you started on eating better during your life change in motion.

3

A Difficult Truth

Making decisions in life is inevitable, but in order to make the best decisions possible, one must be informed. Take time to do your research and get educated on the facts surrounding every decision you face regarding weight loss and better health.

In my journey to become a better, happier, and healthier human being, my decision to have weight-loss surgery was the best decision for me. In many ways, it was a slam dunk. I was deathly afraid of my type 2 diabetes developing into type 1 diabetes and causing more severe health issues.

In my younger years, it scared me to watch my grandmother, a full-blown diabetic, give herself insulin injections. Back then, I really didn't understand what diabetes was all about. As I got older and was diagnosed as pre-diabetic and subsequently a type 2 diabetic, I realized that I needed to educate myself. I researched how the body processes sugar and what the prognosis would be if my condition went untreated or if my behavior didn't change.

People really don't understand the severity of diabetes, and from my experience, I haven't seen that many become overly concerned when told they have diabetes. Contrast that to those who learn they have cancer, which is a serious wake-up call and a scary word—as it should be.

Diabetes, however, when left untreated or unresolved, can cause death just as cancer can, yet our society seems tolerant of the idea that many of our youth are developing diabetes. In fact, I believe people would be outraged and called to action if our youth were developing cancer at the same rate as diabetes caused by obesity.

To reiterate, I am not a medical doctor, but with my experience and the research that I've done, I fear that we are clearly not on the right path and our society is in trouble. We have to take the time to educate ourselves about these health conditions and their causes to make informed decisions with respect to our own health and those of our loved ones. Education is key!

Obesity: The Underlying Problem

We learned early on that for every cause there is an effect. Diabetes is the effect, but the real cause and underlying problem is obesity. According to the National Institutes of Health, more than two-thirds of adults and one-third of children in the United States are overweight or obese. This statement is staggering and should shake you to your core.

If you think the problem can't be any worse, think again. In 2016, the New Mexico Bariatric Center shed more light on the statistics of weight and obesity issues. In the United States, two-to-nine-year-old children account for 17 percent of obesity cases. That's over 5 million children who are obese. In 2014, a study showed that Arkansas, Mississippi, and Ohio had the highest number of obesity cases.

So, why are we seeing this occur? That's a real head-scratcher because we live in the wealthiest country in the world, so how can it be that we see this type of crisis? Well, more than 14 percent of U.S. households have limited access to healthy food and adequate nutrition, and one in ten adults die from being physically inactive.

Unbelievable, right?

People have to start making better choices regarding their health, more specifically when it comes to eating habits and level of physical activity. The mentality that obesity in our country is acceptable or "par for the course" needs to change. We have to get ourselves and our country on the right path toward restored health. I'm sharing my story and experience in hopes that it will encourage anyone facing obesity to make a change for the better regarding their health and happiness.

If you've given up on trying, I'm standing here as living proof that it is possible to set your *life change in motion* and transition from obesity to restored health. If you can make the conscious decision to eat smaller, healthier portions—coupled with increased activity each day—you can help curb these obesity statistics.

Defining Obesity

What is obesity and how is it calculated? This is something you need to know.

When you think of obesity, what comes to your mind? I know—overweight, fat, and heavy people. Yet the term obesity doesn't just describe appearance. It's a medical condition that has severe health effects.

There are different levels of obesity. In medical terms, obesity is defined as having a BMI or body mass index of 30 or higher. Medical professionals measure your BMI, which is a measure of your weight in relation to your height. There are three classes of obesity:

- Class 1 is a BMI between 30-35
- Class 2 is a BMI between 35-40
- Class 3 is a BMI 40 and above

Classes 2 and 3 are known as severe to morbid obesity, and they are often hard to treat with regular diet and exercise. I encourage you to seek out your medical professional who can help you to obtain your BMI. You can also get a good estimate using the following method: take your weight in kilograms, then divide by your height in meters, and divide once again by your height in meters. This will equal your BMI.

In my case, before bariatric surgery, I weighed 320 pounds, or 145 kilos divided by my height of 1.77 meters two times, which gave me a BMI of 46.3, which was definitely morbidly obese.

Today, my current weight is 160 pounds, which is 72 kilos divided by my height of 1.77 meters two times, which equals a BMI of 22.9, which is ideal.

Once you know your BMI and which class you fall in, your medical professional will assess other risk factors you may have and order more blood work to determine if there is any indication of diabetes or other conditions.

Diabetes Facts

According to the Centers for Disease Control and Prevention (CDC), 29.1 million people, or one out of every eleven people, are diagnosed with diabetes, a disease in which blood glucose levels rise above normal. Like I stated before, education is key. I really had to do my research and learn as much as possible about the different types of diabetes.

There is pre-diabetes, type 1 and type 2 diabetes, and gestational diabetes. Pre-diabetes is diagnosed when the blood sugar level is elevated higher than the normal range but not high enough to fall into range for a diabetes diagnosis. Anyone diagnosed with pre-diabetes has a higher likelihood of it evolving into type 2 diabetes.

Simply put, type 1 diabetes was previously called insulin-dependent diabetes mellitus. This type develops when the cells that produce insulin in the pancreas are destroyed. There is no known way to cure this, and it is required that people who suffer from type 1 diabetes have an insulin pump or injections.

Type 2 diabetes, otherwise known as non-insulin dependent diabetes mellitus, accounts for about 90-to-95 percent of all diagnosed cases. Developing type 2 diabetes is usually associated with risk factors such as old age, obesity, family history, and physical inactivity. For some, ethnicity may also contribute to a higher risk of being diagnosed with type 2 diabetes.

Both the U.S. Census Bureau and CDC studies indicate that of those age twenty or older in the U.S. between 2009 and 2012, 15.9 percent of American Indians and Alaska Natives, 13.2 percent of non-Hispanic blacks, 12.8 percent of Hispanics, 9 percent of Asians, and 7.6 percent of non-Hispanic white Americans suffer from diabetes.

Gestational diabetes is another form of this disease, which affects women and is diagnosed during pregnancy. Blood glucose levels are increased and both mother and child require treatment to reduce the risk of further issues. Children born to women diagnosed with gestational diabetes may have a higher risk of childhood or adolescent obesity which may in turn lead to a type 2 diabetes diagnosis.

In my late twenties, I was diagnosed with pre-diabetes. My blood glucose levels, also known as hemoglobin A1C, were higher than the normal range but not high enough to be classified either of the more serious types of diabetes. Health-care professionals will most likely take the time to warn patients that if you are pre-diabetic, you are at a higher risk of developing type 2 diabetes.

A pre-diabetes diagnosis should be taken as a warning that your health is heading down the wrong path. That's how I viewed things. Knowing the situation I faced, I tried to work out and eat right, but pushing myself to do those things was very difficult for me. Since thyroid issues were a part of my family history, my doctor ordered a blood test to ensure that my thyroid was not the cause of my weight issues.

Many are unaware that the thyroid gland controls a great deal in the body, including weight, which is why it's important to seek out your medical professional in order to be completely educated on all your personal health. In my case, my thyroid was normal, yet by age twenty-nine, I was diagnosed with type 2 diabetes. I knew I was in trouble and something had to change.

My point to all this is that diabetes is a serious disease and an area of your health that requires special attention. The implications are grave for our society. Statistics from the National Health and Nutrition Examination Survey estimated that between 2009 and 2012, 15.1 million diabetics were men and 13.4 million were women. In 2011, about 282,000 people who had increased glucose levels in the blood, or hyperglycemia, visited emergency rooms. These people were at least eighteen years old.

This is a crisis. In 2010, among people ages twenty and above, hyperglycemia caused 2,361 deaths. From 2009-2012, of adults aged 18 or over who were diagnosed with diabetes, 71 percent had high blood pressure and 65 percent had high cholesterol. In 2010, hospitalization rates for heart attack patients were 1.8 times higher among twenty-year-olds and above, and hospitalizations for stroke victims were 1.5 times higher.

Other complications caused by diabetes include nerve disease, fatty livers, hearing loss, erectile dysfunction, depression, and pregnancy complications.

Diabetes also affects your eyes. Between 2005 and 2008, adults over forty years old saw a terrible trend. At least 4.2 million people suffered from diabetic retinopathy, which is damage to the blood vessels in the retina, a condition that can cause blindness. The kidneys are not exempt from issues either. Diabetes was listed as the primary cause of kidney failure in 44 percent of new cases in 2011, and 49,677 people of all ages began treatment for kidney failure due to diabetes.

In 2010, about 73,000 lower limb amputations were performed in diabetics twenty years old or older, so diabetes is a disease that must be taken seriously. If you've been diagnosed as pre-diabetic, take immediate action to start your *life change in motion*. Don't wait until the disease gets out of control. It only gets much harder from that point forward.

In my case, at the point where I was diagnosed with type 2 diabetes, my health was already in bad shape. I was obese and suffered from self-image and confidence issues. I was also suffering from depression. And then came the lowest blow when I visited my doctor for a routine physical exam and he asked me if I was an alcoholic.

"Excuse me," I said. "Why are you asking me that?"

"I'll tell you in a minute," he replied. "Do you drink any hard liquor?"

Again, I was taken aback. "Doctor, you don't understand. I don't drink at all." In fact, I had never drunk any alcohol my entire life.

"The reason I'm asking you these questions is because you have a liver condition called fatty liver, normally a condition associated with alcoholism. But since you say you don't drink alcohol, that must mean your fatty liver comes from being severely overweight."

In 2010, diabetes was the seventh-leading cause of death in the United States. Sadly, just over 69,000 death certificates were issued in which diabetes was listed as the cause of death. As with the number of people who currently suffer from diabetes, the number of deaths is likely underreported because there is a vast number of people that are not formally diagnosed.

Diabetes is estimated to cost the United States a total of over $245 billion. In 2012, over $175 billion went to direct medical costs, and close to $70 billion in indirect costs such as disability, work loss, and premature death.

Diabetes is a very serious disease indeed, and that's a very difficult truth for many to accept.

Bariatric Surgery Statistics

The American Society for Metabolic and Bariatric Surgery (ASMBS), in 2016, noted that the total number of people who underwent bariatric surgery was 196,000 people. Of those, 23.1 percent had gastric bypass, 5.7 percent had the adjustable lap band, and 53.8 percent of those had the sleeve gastrectomy. The number of bariatric patients increased from 2011 when 158,000 people elected to have weight loss surgery.

These surgeries are tools to help people get their weight under control and their lives back on track. Many people however, have misconceptions about bariatric surgery and question whether it's possible for any weight that's been lost to be gained back.

The truth is that most people are more likely to keep the weight off and subsequently reduce their risk of death due to diabetes, kidney failure, heart attack, stroke, and so on. This has been the case for me. Of course, there are always other outcomes to surgeries, and it's important to note that each individual situation is unique. Results are dependent on a number of factors, all of which vary.

As with any major, invasive surgical procedure, death is always a possibility. The larger a person is, the more difficult it is to go through bariatric surgery. Data from the ASMBS bariatric survey showed that within thirty days of bariatric surgery, 0.13 percent or about 1 in 1,000 patients died. Still, I feel this number is low in comparison to the number of patients suffering from obesity and the number of deaths from diabetes itself, as stated before. In my case, the benefits outweighed the risks, and today I live a happier, healthier life.

Food Evolution

We need to wake up America! The facts and statistics I've described in this important chapter are really disheartening. Life today is rushed and complicated to the point that we don't take the time to make good choices that will keep us healthy.

The stories I heard my great-grandparents tell of back in their day, there were those of hard work, lots of physical activity, and lots of eating fresh, healthy foods. I'd like to shed light on this topic. I grew up in the early '80's and was fortunate enough to know my great-grandmother Irene. I was also fortunate enough to have my maternal and paternal grandparents for a large part of my childhood.

I can remember walking in to my great-grandmother's humble home and seeing simple food. Today, we might look at that same food and be hesitant to eat it, but let me explain. My great-grandmother had fried pig skin on the table frequently. She would make fresh homemade flour tortillas daily. She would cook only with pork fat, yet she lived to be ninety-two years old and was very healthy until the day she died.

I often wonder: How was she able to stay so healthy? Was it good genes? Was it good diet? It's definitely something to think about.

I've come to the unscientific conclusion that living in her time induced a healthier lifestyle. Back then they raised their own pigs, chickens, goats, and cows, which all fed them. They ate foods that they worked hard to produce themselves. It took hard work to be in the field daily to harvest and nurture their crops. They lived a simple life and rarely went to the grocery store. Most fruits and vegetables were canned at home.

In hindsight, I have a feeling that my great-grandparents, and to some degree my grandparents, ate better than my generation—not because they had access to more food, but the food that they did have was fresh and not full of sugar or preservatives as well as no fake colors and certainly no fake dyes.

You see, having worked in the food industry for over twenty years, I have seen the evolution of food. As our youth get more and more used to eating fast food as a way of life, I often wonder what my great-grandmother would think.

I think . . . in fact, I'm sure that she would not like the food evolution. She ate simple and "clean" because she knew exactly what she was eating, knew where the food came from, and how it was prepared.

4

Phase 1: Mindset Matters

Phase 1 of my *Life Change in Motion* concept deals with the emotional and mental state of mind required to initiate and follow through with making a change to better your health. Here's a great quote from an unknown author regarding change: "You must make a *choice* to take a *chance* or your life will never *change*."

It's so true. If you think about it, everything begins with a choice or decision. You either take the chance or you don't. If you don't take a chance, you stay on the same path as before. If you do accept the risk of taking a chance, then you are taking a chance that the outcome of the change will be either positive or negative.

Let's face it—change is a difficult part of life to accept. But life is always evolving, and each of us should not fear change but rather embrace it. When you opt for making the change to improve your health, your mindset matters! In order to be successful, you will have to stay committed to the choice you've made and dedicated to doing whatever is necessary to see it through until the end.

Key Mindset Elements

From my experience, I discovered that there are several key mindset elements necessary to ensure success in your Life Change in Motion, whether you pursue the bariatric or non-bariatric path.

First, and as I mentioned before, the mindset to accept and embrace change is needed for a higher likelihood of progress. Second, it's important to set specific, measurable, attainable, realistic, and timely (SMART) goals. Third, I believe that positives produce. By this I mean that positive thinking with regards to your health change will yield better results.

Next, it's important to focus forward. Always keep your eye on what's yet to come and remind yourself to only look back when you want to review how much progress you've made. Lastly, in an area I feel is greatly important, is that faith prevails. I believe that if your faith in God is strong, then you will have the inner strength to see your health goals through to the end.

My hope is to be an encouragement to all who read my book and to all whom I come in contact with, be it through email, a phone call, or personal interaction. And

I hope you will reach out to me because I hope to connect with you on a level of humility and love.

Not in One Place

If you were looking to categorize my state of mind in my old life, I would say that I was anxious.

You see, my mindset prior to losing weight was all over the place. The only thing I knew for sure what that I was unhappy with myself. Making the choice to set my life change in motion with weight-loss surgery was a tough decision to make. Not only did this procedure have a huge impact on me, but it affected my family as well.

I made the choice to change, and I made it with a heavy heart, knowing that I might not survive bariatric surgery. That was scary, but at the same time, I felt excitement when thinking about the results and possibilities. Placing myself in a state of mind to move forward was easy yet difficult at the same time. It was easy because I was so ready for this change. I wanted to be thin all my life, but I also wanted to be healthy even more. I now know that I am who I should have been all my life.

Agreeing to undergo surgery was a difficult decision because my response was voluntary. I elected to make this change knowing that it could all go wrong. At the same time, I knew that God had a plan for my life, and if it was time to leave this earth, then it was going to happen no matter what I decided. My biggest fear going into this was that my choice to make this change could affect me negatively for the rest of my life, whether my time was short or long. Another consideration was the impact on my family. I wanted to protect my heart and theirs, but I knew that if I didn't take this step, I would forever be unhappy.

Some may wonder why I didn't just make my life change in motion through dieting and exercise. My response is simple: I felt that I had gone past the point of no return. My health had already sunk into a deep mire and had taken a bad turn for the worse. If I didn't do something—like undergo bariatric surgery—then I wasn't looking at long to live. That's why I felt my decision was right for me. My biggest fear was that I would try my best and not see the result anyway. What kept me going was the encouragement I felt that I would have a second chance to live a better life—and to be a better me!

Here's my advice to you, if you're considering making a life change in motion. First, educate yourself, and then discuss your options with medical professionals. When you think you have all the information you need, follow your heart. Ultimately, you and only you can make these all-important health-care decisions for yourself.

I do not recommend bariatric surgery for teenagers unless it's absolutely medically necessary. My encouragement to anyone out there struggling with weight or self-image issues is that you can be a better person as long as you choose to be. If it means taking drastic steps that include bariatric surgery, then so be it. I urge you to look to the future and strive to be the best person that you were intended to be. Whatever your decision, you must see it through to the very end.

I would like to, for a brief moment, remind everyone that I embraced my decision to have bariatric surgery. My mindset from that point on was amazing, and I believe it's because I was mentally ready to make this change and become whole again.

Since my bariatric surgery, I have done very well, but the one thing that did not go well was having surgery to remove excess skin three-and-a-half years after my original bariatric surgery.

The skin removal part of my journey was one of those things that I expected to go well but didn't. I was unhappy with the hanging skin around my abdomen area and wanted it removed. This was an elective surgery that turned out to be an awful experience.

I should have listened to my gut because two weeks before the surgery, I didn't feel right about undergoing the procedure, which means I didn't have the same positive mindset that I had going into my bariatric surgery. I wish I had listened to my gut, but I set my misgivings aside and had the operation anyway.

I had a tough journey afterward that I wouldn't want to wish upon anyone. That said, I have no complaints about the journey I'm on.

What happened, happened, and there's nothing I can do to change it. I now have the mindset that having the skin removal surgery was a bump in the road to recovery.

A Mindset of Looking Ahead

So where am I today?

I'd say that today I'm a changed man. I know that I live life to the fullest. God has kept me in the palm of His hand and walked with me every step of the way. My life change in motion has taken me from obesity to restored life, from darkness to vibrancy.

My body has changed so much. Now when I see my doctors, they always do blood tests, as they should. When the results come back, they pronounce me as healthy as a child, which is hilarious to me. If they only knew how overjoyed and full of life I feel.

One change that I had to get used to was having a new self-image. Growing up, I was bullied because I was heavyset. Even as an adult I faced bullying and put-down comments and asides, which I never thought would be so prevalent at thirty years old.

Now that I'm a "new Jacob," people who knew me years ago often tell me that they cannot remember me being so overweight or even picture me as the heavy guy I used to be. The most obvious change is my personal appearance, but what they can't see is how my mind has changed. That's almost as important as the weight loss.

I'm here to tell you my life is great. I learned that our spirit has a huge impact and plays a vital role in our lives. You see, we have a body, which is the vessel for our souls, and we have a spirit that lives within our soul. Our body is visible to all, but our souls are not at all visible. Our spirit is something very personal to each of us, and it is truly the only communication tool that we have directly to our Maker.

I'm now in tune with my body, mind, and soul and intend to keep it that way!

5

Phase 2: The Bariatric Process

Let's move on to Phase 2 of my Life Change in Motion Concept, which focuses primarily on the bariatric process.

As I stated previously, making the decision to undergo bariatric surgery should not be taken lightly. Prior to making such a commitment, you have to get informed and know all the facts, which means consulting with your medical professional as my book is not intended to provide medical advice or to take the place of medical advice and treatment from your personal physician.

That said, the information I provide in this section is based on my experience and meant to help you start building your foundation of knowledge with respect to bariatric surgery. There are great resources available online for your benefit. I've included a list of these in an Appendix.

Bariatric surgical procedures are those in which weight loss is induced by restricting the amount of food the stomach can hold. The three most common types of weight loss surgery are:

- adjustable gastric band
- sleeve gastrectomy
- gastric bypass

While there are similarities between these three procedures, there are key differences that are worth noting. It's important that you understand each procedure before selecting the right one for your situation.

Adjustable Gastric Band

The adjustable gastric band, also known as a lap band, is a surgical procedure that can be adjusted or reversed, thus its name. With this procedure, the surgeon places a small ring with an inner inflatable band around the top of your stomach. What this does, in essence, is create a small pouch.

This ring makes you feel full as soon as you start eating. A surgeon can adjust the band by using a circular balloon inside the body that is filled with a solution that can be adjusted larger or smaller, depending on how much weight you want to lose. If the band causes issues that become too big to surmount, it may need to be removed.

There are lower risks of surgical-related problems, but they do exist. As with any procedure, undergoing the operation will require a hospital stay, but this procedure usually requires less time convalescing than the other options. There are no changes to your intestines, but there is a less chance that your body will suffer from vitamin deficiency.

Most likely you will not experience as much weight loss as with gastric bypass or a sleeve gastrectomy, but that doesn't mean that an adjustable gastric band isn't a good option. The adjustable gastric band does require frequent follow-up visits, and there is potential that future issues may arise causing either the necessity for removal of the band or the replacement of certain parts.

Sleeve Gastrectomy

The sleeve gastrectomy procedure will yield greater weight loss than the adjustable band. Just like the adjustable gastric band, there is no change to your intestines.

Sleeve gastrectomy is a procedure in which your surgeon removes most of your stomach, leaving a sleeve-like section that is closed with staples. There are no foreign objects placed in the body and this procedure does not require a long hospital stay.

This method also reduces the amount of food that you can eat and makes you feel full rather quickly. This procedure can affect your gut hormones and remove some of the bacteria that might affect your metabolism and your appetite.

A sleeve gastrectomy is a serious option and must be considered carefully because this procedure cannot be reversed since part of the stomach is removed permanently. This is why many people choose to go with the adjustable lap band. As stated before and most important, the sleeve cannot be reversed. As with any bariatric procedure, you can experience a vitamin deficiency. There is a great chance of acid reflux, and there are also high chances that there could be surgical-related problems.

Gastric Bypass

The third procedure I am highlighting is gastric bypass, also known as the Roux-en-Y. Known as the "gold standard" of weight-loss surgery, this is the procedure that I opted to undergo.

First the surgeon creates a small pouch by stapling your stomach into a pouch in the top or upper section. This will cause you to eat less and feel full very quickly. The surgeon then cuts your small intestine and attaches the lower part directly to your new "pouch."

What this means is that food bypasses most of your stomach, and you absorb less calories from your food. For this reason, I am on a strict vitamin regimen daily, and everyone who chooses gastric bypass must be on a regimented vitamin plan as well. The bypass section is still attached to the main stomach, which allows digestive juices to break down food in the small intestine. The bypass does change your gut hormones or gut bacteria, which most certainly will affect your appetite and metabolic rate.

Gastric bypass patients often have greater weight loss than those who undergo other procedures. As with most weight-loss surgeries, vitamin deficiency is a real issue and must be monitored frequently. This procedure is difficult to reverse, but the possibility for a surgeon to reverse it exists only if found to be medically necessary. In fact, my doctors warned me that gastric bypass was almost impossible to reverse. I was given a stern warning that in major cases of difficulty, the reversal or attempt to reverse gastric bypass can be fatal. As with most surgical procedures, chances of surgical-related issues arising with gastric bypass are significant.

It's important for me to reiterate that I made the best choice for me. I must also mention, as I often do, that any weight loss procedure is a tool and only a tool. The behaviors of any individual must change in order to maintain healthy weight and ensure success in any weight-loss surgical procedure.

Open vs. Laparoscopic Surgery

Over the years, amazing advancements in technology have allowed the health-care industry to introduce new techniques and options in your medical treatment. One of those advancements is an option to have a bariatric procedure done through a laparoscopic approach.

Laparoscopy is a minimally invasive surgery done with the assistance of a video camera and thin instruments. Your medical professional will tell you what options you have, but primarily, if a weight-loss procedure can be completed laparoscopically, most doctors will advise to use that option. This type of procedure is lower in risk and much less invasive. The recovery time is considerably shorter and easier on your body. There is also less scarring with laparoscopic surgery since incisions are smaller, which also reduces the risk of infection dramatically.

While there are noteworthy benefits to using this method, laparoscopic surgery may not be an option for many conditions or in certain situations. For bariatric surgery, some medical professionals may choose to perform open surgery if your obesity level will not allow laparoscopic surgery. Other surgeons feel more comfortable with this traditional approach to surgery since they have trained to operate this way.

The Price to Pay

What are the costs associated with weight-loss surgeries?

On average, the cost of weight-loss surgery can range from $15,000 to $50,000, and many variables go into these figures. While most insurance carriers offer some sort of coverage for bariatric procedures, you may be on the hook for a significant portion of medical and hospital costs.

In my case, I was fortunate that my health insurance covered my gastric bypass procedure because of how high my BMI was.

You must seek consult with your health insurance company to determine what, if any, coverage is offered under your specific plan.

The next question I often hear is this: Does bariatric surgery always work?

Always is an impossible standard. I would reframe the question in this way: Does bariatric surgery work often enough that it's worth the time, effort, and expense?

My answer is an unequivocal yes with the caveat that only if your doctor is in agreement. From my personal experience, gastric bypass has been my lifesaver. I will say, however, that I have heard stories from many people who said the results were not what they expected. Many people lose 15 to 30 percent of their starting weight on average, but depending on which procedure they chose or how dedicated they were to change, they didn't lose as much as they expected.

Bariatric surgery is a tool and that alone. Gastric bypass surgery forced me to break bad eating habits and replace them with eating correctly; that has been my saving grace. I underwent a life change knowing that there was a risk of complications developing, the chance of being stricken with dumping syndrome (a condition in which food, especially sugar, moves from the stomach to the small intestine too quickly), and the possibility of regaining any weight I lost.

In fact, I have met a few people that have gained most, if not all, of their original weight back. For them, they felt the cost was too high or the pain was not worth it. That's not the mindset you should have going in. If you opt for bariatric surgery, hard work, commitment, and dedication are required to experience the best results possible.

Prepping for Surgery

Before surgery, I met with my doctor several times as well as with a dietician, a psychiatrist, and the bariatric surgeon. I went through a series of medical exams and had to endure quite a bit of blood work.

I have never been a smoker so this did not apply to me, but if you smoke, you will have to refrain from lighting up six weeks prior to surgery. A dietician will help you understand how to navigate your new habits after surgery, and a psychologist will help you understand how the changes will affect you mentally. You will also be advised that you should increase your level of activity and exercise regularly.

It's important that you don't underestimate the degree of the transformation your body and mind will make. Following surgery, there were times when I felt like the old me had passed away, which triggered a period of mourning for the person that was no longer me.

Believe me, that was a strange feeling. Even stranger still was looking in the mirror six months after and seeing a new person in my reflection.

But that's what I signed up for, right?

The After Results

After surgery, I had to take time to rest and recover from everything my body had been through. Since walking was encouraged just hours after my procedure, I was up and walking around, albeit very slowly. For the next several weeks, I was limited to a strict liquid diet.

In fact, I can remember the day that I had progressed to the point where I was allowed to have low sodium chicken stock. To me, that was a really great day and a delicious "meal" that I can remember being filling and quite sufficient.

Every person is unique, and every "after" experience will be different. In my case, the weight loss was quick; I lost 50 pounds in the first thirty days of post-surgery. For each month thereafter, I lost an average of 15 pounds per month until the six-month mark, when my weight loss slowed dramatically until I reached my lowest weight of 160 pounds. Over a nine-month span, I lost a total of 160 pounds—half my original weight!

Most people gain some weight back over time, which is normal, but it's a small amount of weight as compared to beforehand—or at least it should be. Moving forward, it was clear to me that my weight loss and future would depend on my level of commitment and dedication to staying on a portion-controlled eating plan, following instructions from my doctors while maintaining a healthy lifestyle.

One of the greatest changes for me—and one of the hardest—was eating out at restaurants. I had to retrain my mind to be health conscious and focus on portion control, eating portion sizes that were sufficient to nourish my body but not overindulge. What I found that works for me was ordering off the children's menu.

The children's menu? Aren't I a little old for kid's fare? Actually, in some restaurants, if you inform them that you have certain dietary restrictions, they will allow you to order from the children's menu. If they don't allow me to do that, then I will order side dishes and choose only the healthiest items, especially at places that don't seem to be health conscious. As a result, I have learned what to order and how to get the best nutritional food at just about any place.

As you can see from my before-and-after photos, the results of losing so much weight made a dramatic difference in my appearance. Losing the weight lifted my self-esteem, but more importantly, I can't tell you what a difference losing that weight has had on how I feel physically, mentally, and spiritually.

The Positive and Negative

Overall, I experienced both positive and negative effects, but for me the positive aspects have outweighed the negative ones by far.

Let's look first at the positive effects.

Like I said, my life change resulted in benefits that I still find overwhelming. From my weight loss surgery, I have experienced a positive health change in:

- high blood pressure, which is now completely normal
- cholesterol levels, which are now completely normal
- type 2 diabetes, which is now gone
- my liver, which is now completely normal
- my sleep patterns, which are now completely normal
- knee and hip pain, which are now gone

My attitude has improved, and my energy levels are as high as I can remember. I couldn't be any happier. If and when you decide to do something about your health, your life change in motion will be unique, and know that results may vary.

I do realize that not everyone will have as great of an experience as I did with weight loss. Still, if you're struggling with weight issues and are finding it hard to carry the burden any longer, I encourage you to set your life change in motion. I recommend weight-loss surgery as an option and encourage you to consult with and seek the blessing of your doctor. But please know that you do not have to undergo weight-loss surgery if you don't absolutely need it or wish to avoid the bariatric route. I chose this path because I was in a life-and-death trap. My BMI was so high, and the risk of me dying at a young age were real and frankly scared the daylights out of me.

As for the negative effects, it's naïve to think you can go through the bariatric process and not experience side effects or some type of negative impact on your body. As with any form of medical treatment, there is always a small—maybe big—chance you could experience an unanticipated result of some sort. For this reason, I went into my life change with eyes wide open and made an objective choice to pursue gastric bypass surgery because the possible positive effects outweighed the negative.

But the choice is yours to make.

So what are the side effects of undergoing bariatric surgery? Some include bleeding or infection in addition to intestinal leaks, diarrhea, blood clots, vomiting, and nausea. After weight-loss surgery, there is a possibility you can develop hernias.

When you choose weight loss surgery, research suggests that your body processes food and absorbs nutrients differently. The body will also absorb alcohol differently, and for that reason it is highly recommended that people *not* drink alcohol after this procedure because an enzyme in the stomach that usually begins to digest alcohol is not there or is greatly reduced.

For this reason and many others, careful consideration of your commitment and dedication to this life change in motion should be taken from the beginning of the decision-making process.

I'm sure you will make the right decision for where you are at this time in your life.

6

Phase 3: Choosing Your Path

No matter how grim your individual situation may seem, it's important to remember you have options—both bariatric and non-bariatric. For either path, take the time to do your research so that you can make an informed decision. Each path has the potential to yield significant results if you stay committed to following your life change in motion through to the end. My goal is to help you by offering the benefit of my experience and the lessons I've learned.

To review, the bariatric path is a surgical option that will assist you in weight loss and getting your health on track. Let me outline these options again:

- The adjustable lap band procedure is where a rubber band-like device is inserted into your body and wrapped around your stomach. The band can be adjusted to allow less food to be consumed, but it can also be opened so that more food can be taken in. (Nobody wants to starve.) The adjustable lap band is a tool that allows the patient to monitor and take in less-than-normal amounts of food.

- The sleeve gastrectomy is a procedure where the stomach is converted into a "sleeve." This means a surgeon must go in and remove a portion of your actual stomach and create a sleeve to reduce food intake.

- Last, there is the Roux-en-Y, or more commonly known as gastric bypass. This is where your stomach is completely separated from your intestine. Your surgeon then creates a small pocket, or pouch, about the size of an egg. This pouch becomes the new stomach where your food will go. However, with such a small "stomach," this makes it difficult to eat large amounts of food, which cuts caloric intake. The pouch also lacks the stomach's ability to absorb all nutrients from your food; therefore, you will have to be on a vitamin regimen for the remainder of your life.

The side effects for each of these procedures are similar. If you eat too much food or sugar, or eat too fast, you can experience a "dumping" syndrome. This, believe me, is no fun at all and causes great abdominal pain as well as bouts of vomiting and diarrhea.

Remember, each of these procedures is just a tool that requires discipline in order to realize and maintain good results. The discipline part is tough for us because we each have a free will, which means we can choose to make choices that work for or against our own good. Some choices are easy, but in the area of losing weight, these choices become much more difficult.

For instance, the choice to eat less is one of the hardest to make. Those who can't discipline themselves or "give in" will suffer the circumstances, as in experiencing the dumping syndrome. Another side effect that sleeve gastrectomy and gastric bypass patients don't think about is that a lack of discipline means they could retrain their new stomach to hold more and more food, thus causing minimal weight loss and potential weight gain in the future.

The bariatric path is not for everyone, and surgery may not be a viable option for many, especially if there are financial considerations or lack of adequate insurance. Please allow me to assure you that you have the option to choose the non-bariatric path to weight loss.

Whatever direction you decide to go regarding weight loss, you should consult your physician. If you choose to go on the non-bariatric path, your physician will advise you to get on a regular exercise program that will increase your level of activity and help you to help burn calories.

It's important to consider your limits and abilities. Remember that you don't climb the highest mountain right away. You make progress up the hill by getting in better shape and building up your strength and endurance. Over time, you can work your way up to a more aggressive exercise regimen.

You should also follow a sensible meal plan. In fact, the biggest thing I've learned is that everyone should be following a small, portion-controlled eating plan. Following this eating schedule is important and impactful because the number of calories you take in is just as important whether you're on the non-bariatric path or the bariatric path. Therefore, the portioning of food is crucial for success in any life change in motion.

I'll share more about my Portion Your Plate eating plan in Chapter 9.

What to Consider

When you are considering any life change in motion, you must first consider the current state of your health. The amount of weight you need to lose to reach your ideal healthy state is significant in helping you to determine your path.

For example, if you need to lose 20 pounds, then choosing a bariatric procedure, or more specifically gastric bypass, may not be the best option to take to accomplish your goal. In fact, most doctors will not perform gastric bypass surgery unless you are extremely obese, meaning you have a BMI above 40.

I discussed previously in Chapter 3 about what the BMI is and how it's calculated. Your doctor can help you figure out what your BMI is, and only a medical professional can give you accurate numbers. You can get an estimate of your BMI from tools commonly used in gyms by fitness trainers, but the actual BMI test is given by a trained medical professional.

Consider this: Your health and overall wellness are too important to leave in the hands of anyone other than your primary care physician. It's also important to be open and honest with yourself about your eating lifestyle. If you're in the habit of eating fast foods, drinking sugary drinks, and consuming alcoholic beverages, then you're in for a rude awakening. You will and must be committed to changing your poor eating and drinking habits in order for you to be successful following either the bariatric or non-bariatric path.

Getting into good eating and drinking habits is essential to weight loss and improving your overall state of health. It's my contention, through my experiences, that you can live a happy and healthy life by eating portioned, wholesome foods, and by enjoying refreshingly simple, clean, and healthy beverages.

Important Steps to Take

Whichever path you decide to take there are certain aspects to be considered and steps you should take to begin the process. You may see similarities and differences in each of these paths. At any rate, once you've decided on your route to losing weight, these steps will help guide you along the way.

It's important to remind you that these steps were ones I used in my journey, and they may not be for everybody. You may find that along your way, your steps may not be exactly as mine and that's alright. I am not a physician, a dietician, or a nutritionist. I am just someone who has been where you are standing and someone who embarked on the journey you're about to embark on.

What I'm trying to do is provide encouragement and lessons from my experiences to help make your transition into your life change in motion somewhat easier.

Consider this graph on the steps you need to take:

Bariatric Path	Non-Bariatric Path
Seek medical advice	Seek medical advice
State of health assessment	State of health assessment
BMI calculation	BMI calculation
Blood work	Blood work
Cholesterol count	Cholesterol count
Blood pressure	Blood pressure
Blood sugar, A1C	Blood sugar, A1C
Other tests specified by physician	Other tests specified by physician
Get informed	Begin an exercise regimen.
Research procedures	Start small and slow and
Consider financial implications	increase as you go.

Decide which procedure is right for you	Get a friend or family member to help you stay encouraged and accountable
Mental health evaluation	Portion your plate! Start by cutting portion sizes in half, then track your daily food intake and count your calories.
Schedule your procedure	Reward yourself for any successes
Pre-surgical preparation Day of surgery Recovery	
Post-surgical lifestyle changes Follow exercise and dietary restrictions Portion your plate! Monitor food intake Count calories	
Reward yourself for any successes	

Which Is Your Path?

The choice you make is an extremely personal decision based on the state of your health, your mindset, and your physician's recommendations. There are many factors involved, but ultimately the decision rests with each of you.

I chose bariatric surgery mainly because of the perceived benefits to my health. But I have to be honest and disclose that there was a very personal emotional side to my decision. During my life, I had some eye-opening moments that destroyed any confidence I had in myself and contributed to my low self-image. I did not feel good about who I was or how people looked at me.

I wouldn't be surprised if you feel the same way or had the same experiences. No one suffering from weight control issues, no matter how heavy or obese, is helped when they are told they are fat or made to feel ashamed about their weight and appearance.

I was hooked on soda, so when people told me that drinking soda pop was bad, I chose not to listen. That didn't motivate me to stop sipping sodas. The same holds true with losing weight. No one responds well to bullying or being told they're fat and will always be fat if they keep porking out.

You see, anyone dealing with weight control issues is hurting already. They *know* they're too heavy, and quoting studies on diabetes or cardiovascular disease only exasperates the situation and causes a negative effect. Anything you say to friends in a similar situation can be taken wrongly since their mindset is already weakened and could lead them to hurt themselves or push them into a dark depression. It's always best to encourage a change through healthy foods and exercise, but your words must be chosen in a helpful way.

In my workplace, the franchise owner once had a wealthy investor join our company. One particular day when I was touring him and his wife around the cafes, I offered to get them some breakfast. Remember that I have always been in the food business, and hospitality comes natural to me.

The husband and wife both declined my offer of breakfast, but twenty minutes later, I offered to get them some food, to be polite. My offer was met with a derogatory comment from the husband that I will never forget: "No thanks, I don't want to look like you."

I was crushed, embarrassed, and humiliated by his comment. If I could have crawled into the smallest corner of the world, I would have.

On a separate occasion, I was met by a very large person at the doorstep of one of my restaurants. I looked at him, and he looked right back at me. It was me! When I saw my reflection in the glass door, I suddenly realized what I had become.

The person I saw was someone I knew but someone who never accepted who he was. This was an eye-opening moment that made me realize I did not love myself enough to take good care of myself. This was a huge defining moment and one that pushed me to initiate my life change in motion. I realized that I had control over that guy in the glass reflection.

My advice for anyone who's struggling with weight issues is this: You must come to the realization that you're at point where you don't want to be. If you feel like you've hit rock bottom, then you've likely reached that point.

You also have to accept the fact that you are willing to change and more importantly that you're *ready* to change. Embracing the idea of change and committing to seeing it through to the end is the first of many steps. For bariatric procedures, the pre-surgery mental evaluation will help ensure you are ready for any challenges you may face. If you choose the non-bariatric path, I recommend you take the same steps anyway. You should still seek advice from your physician, a dietician, and a psychologist.

Get into the mindset of preparing yourself for change. Change itself can be great, but normally it's resisted for a long time as there are few people who like change. Embrace change and embrace yourself on your weight-loss journey.

If you go the non-surgical route, you know that weight loss will be hard, take longer, and require a lot of discipline. At the end of your journey, all that matters is that you achieve your desired results.

The methods to the weight loss may be different, but the effects on the body, mind, and soul are the same. Either path is sure to be a huge challenge, but I know firsthand that any hurdles can be overcome because when you want something bad enough, you will make it happen.

What Made Sense to Me

I've been told many times that I took the easy route when I underwent gastric bypass surgery. Let me assure you, there was nothing, and I do mean NOTHING, easy about the route I chose. I endured great pain and heartache, maybe more so if I had lost weight the traditional non-bariatric way.

I've often asked myself why I decided upon the bariatric route. My honest answer is that I felt in my heart that my life depended on it. I had come from a long line of family members who suffered from diabetes. When I was diagnosed with type 2 diabetes along with high blood pressure and high cholesterol, I knew my prognosis was grim. I had to do something, or I would die an early death.

Is my thought process—that I could die—for everyone who suffers from obesity? The answer is no! There is not a one-size-fits-all option for weight control, and it certainly is important to know it's not the "easy way out" of your obesity problems. After being unsuccessful in other methods to get my weight under control, I was at the end of the line. I needed a boost in the right direction, and bariatric surgery gave me that boost.

So the question I have for you is this: Does bariatric surgery make sense to you?

You can only answer that all-important question, in consultation with your health-care professional. Your success solely depends on your actions before choosing this method *and* the weeks, months, and years following the procedure.

Bariatric surgery has to truly become a new lifestyle for you. And it can, especially after you ask yourself one more key question: Are you worth it?

Sure, you are, just as I thought I was worth it. And since you're worth it, isn't that a good enough reason to go for it?

7

Phase 4: Moving Forward in Your Journey

While Phase 3 focuses on providing information regarding the possible paths to achieve weight loss and getting control of your health, this phase focuses on the what's next for you *after* you've submitted to bariatric surgery or made a major change in your lifestyle by cleaning up your diet and getting on an exercise program.

Either way, you're at the beginning of your new journey. In the very near future, your body will transform, but so will your mind. Life change in motion has begun, so this is not the time to second-guess your decision but to press forward until you reach your goal. But you need to know that your life change in motion is constantly evolving, and it will take some time to truly understand and accept the new you. Moving forward means shifting your focus to embracing and maintaining your restored health.

Your Body Changes

One main way your life change transforms you is your appearance—the way you look to others. After all, you should lose a good amount of weight once you embark on a path. Adjusting to how you feel and see yourself, as well as how others see you, can take some time.

Even after I lost 160 pounds, I still pictured myself as a fat, heavy person, and I have to admit that there are times today when I feel like a heavy person. This is why it's also a great reason to follow your doctor's orders when thinking about bariatric surgery. The mental evaluation will help you to be ready for everything that will come at you during your life change in motion.

You can expect family members, friends, and work colleagues to express shock when they see the new you—especially if the last time they saw you was months earlier. I am five years out from my surgery and weight loss, and still to this day I have people tell me I look great or otherwise compliment me on my weight loss. People who have not seen me in a long time still remember the "old" me, which is why it can be a little strange hearing positive comments. For as long as I can remember, I listened to mean, cutting remarks and felt the negative thoughts about my appearance.

That's going to change now.

In time, you'll be able to start accepting compliments more and more. That's what I had to learn. You see, as a child I had extremely high self-esteem but that disappeared during my adolescent years when the pounds piled on my frame. Now that I've changed through my life change in motion from losing so much weight, my self-esteem has returned. I predict that you'll feel a *lot* better about yourself when the pounds melt away.

Another great change you'll experience is a significant increase in your energy. You'll feel absolutely great when you're not feeling weighted down and tired all the time. I haven't felt this energized since I was a child, and the extra fuel in my tank has helped me increase my daily productivity at work and in my home life.

Your Mind Changes

You probably already know this, but it bears repeating: You will not be able to walk into a hospital one day, get a surgical procedure done, and go home a new person. Or, if you choose the non-bariatric path, you can't expect immediate results.

Not only will your transformation take time and patience, but it will be literally the hardest thing you've ever done in your life.

For me, the hard work really started thirty days *before* my surgery when I successfully completed the pre-surgery classes that Kaiser Permamente required. It's likely that if you choose a different health care facility or clinic, you will be required to complete a similar process so that you're ready and willing to accept changes to your body and its physical appearance.

But as I've said before, change is usually resisted, and I believe that a greater percentage of success in your life change in motion will be a result of your willingness to allow your mind to change. You'll have to learn to let go of what was hurting and hindering you from experiencing a healthy, happy life.

Yes, I'm speaking of bad habits you'll have to give up. I had to learn to eat again, the right way. I had to give up foods I loved such as red meat, pork, soda and more—all in exchange for a healthier, restored self. I also started exercising on a regular schedule.

Then there's the mental side. Mostly, though, I'm referring to letting go of the negativity, guilt, and deep emotions you have inside that you are holding on to tightly. In order for your mind to move forward, you have to forgive yourself. My life change in motion allowed me to get into a mental state of renewal. I had to learn to live again, a lifestyle without shame for who I am.

Not only that, I had to learn to love again. Not to love just anyone, but to love myself! Yes, I had to learn to love *me* again, and in turn, now I can share that love with others.

Moving Toward a New Life

In my experience with bariatric surgery, it took time to heal—close to a year. Prior to bariatric surgery, I was broken inside and out. Post-bariatric surgery, I saw my stitches and scars.

In a way I was broken again, but this time in a good way. Why do I say that? Because I was on the way to becoming whole again.

Today I still bear scars on my abdomen. These scars are mine. I own them, and I embrace them. They represent the pain and the tears of my life change in motion so I could, in essence, re-build myself.

My self-esteem, self-confidence, and self-image have all been refurbished. Sure, there were bumps in my path, and I had to overcome body shame and grief about how poor my health was. After surgery, I was shameful that I had to make such a dramatic turnaround, but I willingly made drastic changes for the better. I grieved post-surgery for the person that I lost. The old me died. In some strange way, I missed my old self, but I realized that I didn't want to trade in who I had become.

The next segments in life have been a blessing. To hear people praise my weight loss and hear how good I look has been a great feeling. When I would hear mean or nasty comments about my weight in the past, I would badly want to hear good things about myself. Now I get nothing but positive comments, which lift my spirits, but you know what? It truly doesn't matter because through the journey I've been on, I've learned to only care about what I think of myself.

Don't Be Broken

My choice to initiate my life change in motion via the bariatric path was exactly that—my choice. As for you, the choice is yours to make, bariatric vs. non-bariatric. But once you make the choice, please know that you must own it from beginning to end.

If your choice to lose weight does not include bariatric surgery, you still will bear scars. Your steps will be similar and your stages somewhat the same. Regardless of the path, please allow my story to inspire you in your weight loss journey but also in other areas of your life.

Listen, we are all broken in some way. My story of how I re-built myself will hopefully show you that you can rebuild any area of your life, at any stage.

Journey Moves Forward

My life change in motion journey has taken me from morbid obesity and someone headed for an early demise to a fully healthy and restored state of life. As you move forward in your journey, I'm confident that you will live a healthy life and adopt great habits, and not just eating habits. In next steps in life, never allow anyone to make you feel less than who God intended you to be.

My journey is still moving forward, and as I have stated a few times, life change in motion is constantly evolving and actually never-ending. I pray that sharing my journey and experience with bariatric surgery will inspire you to set your weight-loss life change in motion whether via bariatric or non-bariatric path.

No matter what route you take, be sure to eat healthy and portion-controlled servings. You'll learn more about portion-control after I share my recipes in the next chapter.

Please know that this is only the beginning of what I'll be sharing with the world. Let me assure you that there will be more to come!

8

Kitchen Basics and Recipes

It's time to get basically basic.

In the world today, where everything is so complicated, we often get tired just thinking about what we have to do—especially when it comes to cooking. A lot of people will do anything *not* to cook, which is reflected in the restaurant industry statistics. These days, families are eating out at restaurants more than ever before, continuing a trend that has seen year-to-year increases since the 1950s.

From the crack of dawn to late-night runs, between 20 and 25 percent of the U.S. population pass through a drive-through lane or line up at a fast-food counter to order something quick and tasty *every day*. (And 7 percent of the U.S. population goes to McDonald's every day as well.) With nearly 300,000 quick-serve restaurants to choose from, Americans fork over more money on burgers, burritos, and bacon-topped sandwiches each year than what we spend on higher education, new cars, and computers combined.

All that being said, I have a few theories to share. Back in the 1950s, adult women were more likely to be married and homemakers with children underfoot. The advantages to having Mom at home are vast. The nutritional value in each meal was measured by a shared meal with family members. She prepared meals that were fresh from foods that were free of preservatives, added colors, added sugars, and hormones.

Moms cooked because it was too expensive to eat out and because the fast food restaurant industry was in its infancy. With a one-income household, one of Mom's big jobs was feeding the family on a budget, so she had put some thought into the meals she cooked. Today, however, fast food meals are much more affordable, and with many mothers in the workforce and too pooped to cook, the family ends up visiting their favorite fast-food restaurants and local eateries several times a week, if not more.

In my quest for weight loss, one of the things I learned is the value of eating a meal at home, which not only saves you plenty of money, but also enriches the family with conversation and closeness—as long as the cell phones are left off the table. Eating at home will provide you with a level of knowledge to what you and your kids are consuming, especially from a perspective of nutrition and portion size.

If eating out is a regular occurrence in your household, I urge you to get back into the kitchen and start cooking up a storm. Well, maybe not a storm, but with some planning and some effort, your efforts will be handsomely rewarded.

To assist you, I have put together a list of basic necessities for your household kitchen. The first list are kitchen tools required to create any basic meal. The second list provides healthier substitutions and alternatives to meal items that may not be so healthy.

And finally, I present delicious, gourmet, and portion-controlled recipes with fresh and healthy ingredients.

Ready to get started? Good . . . now roll up those sleeves!

RECIPE SECTION

Drinks

Honey Mandarin Hot Tea
Pomegranate & Blackberry Hot Tea
Honey Ginger Lemon Tea
Blueberry & Watermelon Chiller
Georgia Peach & Strawberry Smoothie
Slim Pina Colada
Refreshing Pink Lemonade
Fresh Mint Lemon-Limeade

Honey Mandarin Hot Tea

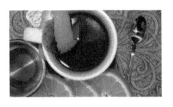

Prep Time: 5 Min.
Yield: 5 Servings

Ingredients	Amount	Measure	Have It	Need Qty
Filtered Water	5	cups		
Black Tea Leaves	5	bags (1oz per cup)		
Honey	1	tablespoon		
Mandarin Orange	1/2	juice & zest		
Filtered Water	5	cups		

Instructions

1. In a tea kettle, bring 5 cups filtered water to a rolling boil.
2. Once hot, turn off the burner and add 5 tea bags.
3. Cover and allow to steep for 3 minutes.
4. Juice 1 mandarin orange for every 2 cups of tea. Add the zest of 1 mandarin orange.
5. Pour and serve.

Pomegranate &
Blackberry Hot Tea

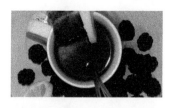

Prep Time: 5 Min.
Yield: 5 Servings

Ingredients	Amount	Measure	Have It	Need Qty
Filtered Water	5	cups		
Black Tea Leaves	2	bags (1oz per cup)		
Fresh Blackberries	1	oz per cup		
Pomegranate Seed	1	oz per cup		
Fresh Lemon	1	teaspoon		

Instructions

1. Bring water to a rolling boil in a tea pot.

2. Once hot, add tea leaves or bags.

3. Steep tea leaves/bags for 4 minutes.

4. Pour into a cup and add a splash of lemon.

5. Add a few fresh blackberries and pomegranate seeds.

6. Add some lemon zest and garnish with a lemon slice.

7. Enjoy!

Honey Ginger Lemon Hot Tea

Prep Time: 5 Min.
Yield: 6 Servings

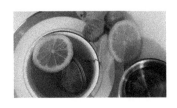

Ingredients	Amount	Measure	Have It	Need Qty
Filtered Water	5	cups		
Chamomile	4	bags (1oz per cup)		
Fresh ginger root	1/2	teaspoon		
Honey	3	tablespoons		
Lemon	1	splash		

Instructions

1. In a tea pot, bring water to a rolling boil.
2. Add 4 bags of chamomile tea. Allow to steep covered for 4 minutes.
3. Peel some ginger root and shred it in the pot.
4. Add 3 Tbsp. honey to the pot.
5. Add a splash of lemon and the zest.
6. Serve and Enjoy!

Blueberry & Watermelon Chiller

Prep Time: 5 Min.
Yield: 6 Servings

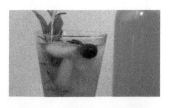

Ingredients	Amount	Measure	Have It	Need Qty
Filtered Water	4	cups		
Fresh blueberries	1/3	cup		
Fresh watermelon	2	cups		
rosemary	1	sprig		
coconut sugar	3	tablespoons		

Instructions

1. In a blender, blend watermelon chunks until liquefied.
2. In a pitcher, add water, liquefied watermelon, coconut sugar, and fresh blueberries.
3. Mix well.
4. Add ice.
5. Serve divided in 6 glasses.
6. Garnish each with fresh mint and rosemary sprig as desired. Enjoy.

Georgia Peach & Strawberry Smoothie

Prep Time: 15 Min.
Yield: 6 Servings

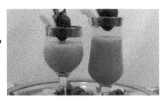

Ingredients	Amount	Measure	Have It	Need Qty
Fresh strawberries	2	cups		
Frozen peaches	2	cups		
Coconut water	2	cups		
Ice	3	cups		

Instructions

1. In a vita mix blender, add strawberries, frozen peaches, coconut water, and ice.
2. Blend on high for 45 seconds.
3. Serve and enjoy

Slim Pina Colada

Prep Time: 10 Min.
Yield: 6 Servings

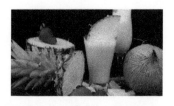

Ingredients	Amount	Measure	Have It	Need Qty
Toasted coconut	1/2	cup		
Crushed pineapple	1	cup		
Pineapple juice	1	cup		
Coconut mil	1 3/4	cup		
Vanilla extract	2	tablespoons		
Coconut sugar	1/3	cup		
Ice	3	cups		

Instructions

1. In a blender, add toasted coconut, crushed pineapple, pineapple juice, coconut milk, vanilla, coconut sugar, and ice.
2. Blend on High until smooth.
3. Divide and pour into six tall glasses.
4. Garnish each with fresh pineapple. Enjoy!

Refreshing Pink Lemonade

Prep Time: 15 Min.
Yield: 6 Servings

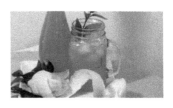

Ingredients	Amount	Measure	Have It	Need Qty
Filtered water	6	cups		
Maraschino cherry juice	1	cup		
Lemons	6	juice and zest		
Stevia	3	packets		
Fresh mint	4	sprigs		

Instructions

1. In a large pitcher add filtered water, juice from a jar of maraschino cherries, lemon juice & zest, and stevia.
2. Mix well.
3. Add fresh mint.
4. Serve ice cold.

Fresh Mint Lemon Limeade

Prep Time: 10 Min.
Yield: 6 Servings

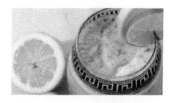

Ingredients	Amount	Measure	Have It	Need Qty
Filtered water	6	cups		
Fresh lemons	4	juice and zest		
Fresh limes	6	juice and zest		
Fresh mint	3	tablespoons		
Coconut nectar	1/3	cup		

Instructions

1. In a blender, add 1 cup of water, fresh lemon juice and zest, fresh lime juice and zest, 3 tbsp. mint, and coconut nectar.
2. Blend until the mint is well incorporated.
3. In a large pitcher, add the mixture and the rest of the filtered water.
4. Add ice and for garnish, a slice each of lemon and lime.

Breakfast

Egg White Omelet
Golden Raisin & Maple Oatmeal
Farm Fresh Eggs

Egg White Omelet

Prep Time: 5 Min.
Yield: 1 Servings

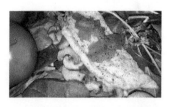

Ingredients	Amount	Measure	Have It	Need Qty
Fresh eggs	2	eggs		
Spinach	1/2	cup		
Tomato	1/2	tomato		
Mushrooms	1/3	cup		
smoked gouda	2	oz		
olive oil	1	teaspoon		
salt & pepper		desired amount		

Instructions

1. Prep veggies ahead of time. Chop the tomatoes using a small dice. Chop the mushrooms using a small dice.
2. In a small mixing bowl, crack 2 fresh eggs and remove the yolks. Add salt & pepper.
3. In a small sauté pan, add a small drizzle of olive oil.
4. Sauté the tomatoes, mushrooms and spinach.
5. Whisk the egg whites and add to the veggies.
6. Cook for 1 minute on LOW heat. Turn and add the smoked gouda cheese.
7. Serve on a bed of fresh spinach.

Golden Raisin &
Maple Oatmeal

Prep Time: 5 Min.
Yield: 4 Servings

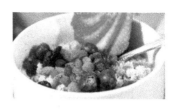

Ingredients	Amount	Measure	Have It	Need Qty
Raw oatmeal	12	oz		
golden raisins	1/2	cup		
Fresh blueberries	13	cup		
Cinnamon	1/2	teaspoon		
Coconut sugar	4	teaspoons		
Pecans	1/4	cup		
Coconut/Almond milk	1/2	cup		
Maple syrup	1	oz		

Instructions

1. Bring 2 cups of water to a boil. Add a pinch of salt.
2. Once water is boiling, bring down to a simmer and add the oats.
3. Add the coconut sugar and dried golden raisins.
4. Cover oats and turn off the burner. Leave covered for 3 minutes.
5. Serve for 4 and top the oatmeal with fresh blueberries, pecans, add a small drizzle of maple syrup and a dash of cinnamon.
6. Enjoy…Breakfast is served.

Farm Fresh Eggs

Prep Time: 10 Min.
Yield: 1 Servings

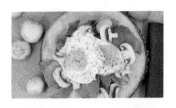

Ingredients	Amount	Measure	Have It	Need Qty
Fresh eggs	2	eggs		
Spinach	1/2	cup		
Mushrooms	1	cup		
Cherry tomatoes	1/2	cup		
Olive oil	1	teaspoon		
Butter	1	teaspoon		

Instructions

1. On medium low heat, heat up 1 tsp. olive oil and ½ tsp. butter.
2. Crack 2 fresh eggs and move the pan around a bit to get the white of the egg to move around.
3. Cook until the white of the egg is firm and serve over fresh raw veggies.
4. Add salt & pepper as desired.

Lunch

Mini Avocado Tea Sandwiches
Crab Tree Tacos
Turkey Burger Sliders

Mini Avocado
Tea Sandwiches
Prep Time: 15 Min.
Yield: 4 Servings

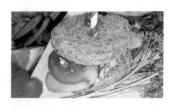

Ingredients	Amount	Measure	Have It	Need Qty
Fresh Haas avocado	2	avocados		
Whole grain bread	8	slices		
Fresh parsley	4	tablespoons		
Cucumber	1/2	cup		
Red onion	1/3	cup		
Fresh garlic	2	cloves		
Feta cheese	4	oz		
Lemon	1	lemon		

Instructions

1. Prep the veggies ahead of time. Chop the cucumber into small pieces. Dice the red onion into small fine pieces. Chop the garlic and parsley.
2. Peel avocados and remove pits. Place avocado in small mixing bowl.
3. Add garlic, onion, and parsley and mix well. Add a splash of lemon to prevent browning.
4. On a cutting board, place the whole grain bread.
5. Spread avocado mixture onto each slice of bread.
6. Top with feta cheese, cucumber and another slice of bread.

Crab Tree Tacos

Prep Time: 25 Min.
Yield: 4 Servings

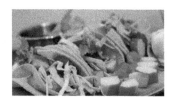

Ingredients	Amount	Measure	Have It	Need Qty
White corn tortillas	8	tortillas		
Shredded cabbage	1/2	head		
Fresh or imitation crab	4	cups		
Cilantro	4	tablespoons		
Canned crushed tomato	1	16oz can		
White onion, diced	1	onion		
Jalepeño, diced	2	peppers		
Fresh garlic	4	cloves		
Kosher salt	1/2	tablespoon		

Instructions

1. Boil the crab meat for 3 minutes, then chop into cubes or shred.
2. Heat corn tortillas on a hot plate.
3. Double stack the corn tortillas and add 2 tsp. crab meat to each one.
4. Add shredded cabbage.
5. Add Salsa Fresca. Add cilantro, if desired.
6. Serve.

Salsa Fresca

1. In a food processor, add canned crushed tomatoes, ½ diced white onion, diced jalapenos, diced fresh garlic, and salt.
2. Blend for 15 seconds or until desired consistency.
3. Place in a serving bowl and serve.

Turkey Burger Sliders

Prep Time: 20 Min.
Yield: 6 Servings

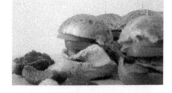

Ingredients	Amount	Measure	Have It	Need Qty
Fresh ground turkey	1	pound		
whole grain minibuns	6	buns		
Butter lettuce	1	head		
Red onion	1	onion		
Tomatoes	2	tomatoes		
Organic Ketchup	6	oz		
Dijon Mustard	6	oz		
Cornichons	1	jar		
Garlic powder	1	teaspoon		
Worcestershire	2	teaspoons		
Salt & pepper		as desired		

Instructions

1. Wash butter lettuce well and peel ahead of time.

2. Slice the vine ripened tomatoes & red onion 1/8 in. thick.

3. In a mixing bowl, add the ground turkey, garlic powder, ½ tsp. salt, Worcestershire sauce, and some fresh ground pepper. Mix without over mixing the meat. Make small 2 oz. patties.

4. In a skillet, lightly brush olive oil. Cook on medium heat for 6-8 minutes until thoroughly cooked. It is best to cook poultry all the way through. *Undercooking meats and poultry is not recommended.

Assembly

1. Once turkey burger patties are cooked, remove them from the skillet and allow them to rest for 5 minutes under aluminum foil.

2. In the same skillet, wipe with paper towel to remove excess oil. Toast each bun for 2 minutes or until lightly toasted (as desired).

3. Place the lettuce, tomato, onion, and patties on the buns, condiments on the side.

Salads - Sides - Soups

Classic Caesar Salad
Farm Beets and Spinach Salad
Grains & Greens Salad
Southwest BBQ Chicken Salad
Simply Sensational Blueberry Salad
Veggie Kabob
Balsamic Brussel Sprouts & Cherry Tomatoes
Health Conscious Deviled Eggs
Farm Fresh Vegetable Stew

Classic Caesar Salad

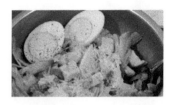

Prep Time: 35 Min.
Yield: 8 Servings

Ingredients	Amount	Measure	Have It	Need Qty
Fresh eggs	4	1/2 per salad		
Hearts of romaine	8	cups		
Boiled skinless chicken breast	4	cups		
Romano cheese	4	tablespoons		
Chicken stock	4	cups		
Greek yogurt	1/2	cup		
Low fat sour cream	1/2	cup		
Anchovy paste	1	tablespoon		
Fresh garlic	2	teaspoons		
Onion powder	1/2	teaspoon		
Fresh lemon	1	juice & zest		

Instructions

Dressing
1. In a medium mixing bowl, add Greek yogurt, low-fat sour cream, anchovy paste, fresh minced garlic, onion powder, lemon juice and zest.
2. Using a wire whisk, mix all ingredients together and serve on the side of the salad.

Chicken
1. In a medium sauce pan, bring 4 cups of low-sodium chicken stock to a boil. Add the skinless, boneless chicken and cook for 30 minutes.
2. Once the chicken is cooked, cool and chop into cubes for the salad.

Salad
1. Chop the hearts of romaine into 1 inch by 1 inch pieces.
2. Shred Romano cheese and add to salad.
3. Top the salad with the cooked chicken.
4. Add boiled egg to the side for added protein.
5. Serve with dressing on the side and enjoy

Farm Beets & Spinach Salad

Prep Time: 15 Min.
Yield: 12 Servings

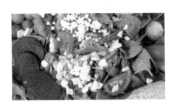

Ingredients	Amount	Measure	Have It	Need Qty
Fresh spinach	6	cups		
Tomatoes	2	tomatoes		
Fresh corn	2	ears		
English cucumber	1	cucumber		
Feta cheese	8	oz		
Red roasted beets	3	beets		
Champagne vinegar	3	tablespoons		
Olive oil	1/2	cup		
Dijon mustard	1	tablespoon		
Lemon	1	lemon	-	
Salt	1/2	teaspoon		
Pepper		as desired		

Instructions

1. In a large salad bowl, place spinach.
2. In a separate medium mixing bowl, whisk the olive oil, Dijon mustard, and champagne vinegar, set aside.
3. Chop tomatoes, cucumbers, red bell peppers.
4. Slice beets and remove corn from ear.
5. Top spinach with vegetables and feta cheese.
6. Serve with dressing on the side.
7. Season with lemon, salt and pepper as desired.

Grains & Greens Salad

Prep Time: 25 Min.
Yield: 4 Servings

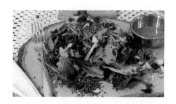

Ingredients	Amount	Measure	Have It	Need Qty
Field greens	4	cups		
Fresh carrots	1	cup		
Quinoa	6	oz		
Raw sliced almonds	1/3	cup		
Raisins	1/2	cup		
White wine vinegar	3	tablespoons		
Apple juice	1/3	cup		
Dijon mustard	1	tablespoon		
Lemon	1	lemon		
Salt & pepper		as desired		

Instructions

1. In a small bowl, place raisins and add 1/3 cup of apple juice to re-hydrate. This will take about 15-20 minutes.
2. In a small mixing bowl, add white wine vinegar, Dijon mustard, the juice of 1 lemon and the zest.
3. Whisk until completely incorporated. Add salt and pepper to taste.
4. In a large bowl, place field greens.
5. Shred carrots and place on top of field greens.
6. Add the cooked ancient grains or quinoa.
7. Top the salad with the raisins and almonds.
8. Serve and enjoy!

Southwest BBQ Chicken Salad

Prep Time: 45 Min.
Yield: 8 Servings

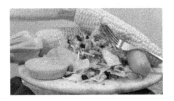

Ingredients	Amount	Measure	Have It	Need Qty
Hearts of romaine	2	hearts		
Fresh corn	2	ears		
Black beans	12	oz		
Parmesan cheese	4	oz		
Chicken breast	2	breasts		
Scallions	6	scallions		
Chicken stock	4	cups		
Greek yogurt	1/2	cup		
Low fat sour cream	1	cup		
Organic Ketchup	1/2	cup		
Worcestershire	6	tablespoons		
Onion powder	1/2	tablespoon		
Garlic powder	1/2	tablespoon		
Red chile powder	1	tablespoon		

Instructions

Dressing

1. In a medium bowl, whisk Greek yogurt, low-fat sour cream, organic ketchup, Worcestershire, onion powder, garlic powder, and red chile powder. Set aside until salad is assembled.

Chicken

1. In a medium sauce pan, bring 4 cups of low-sodium chicken stock to a boil. Add the boneless, skinless chicken and cook for 30 min.
2. Once the chicken is cooked, remove and shred chicken while warm.
3. Save some of the red chile powder from the dressing and add 1 Tsp. to the chicken to season. Add salt to taste.

Salad

1. Chop the hearts of romaine into 1 inch by 1 inch pieces.
2. Shred parmesan cheese and add to salad.
3. Top the salad with the cooled chicken.
4. Remove corn from cob and sauté in a medium sauté pan for 1 minute.
5. Add a can of cooked black beans.
6. Chop scallions and add to the top of the salad.

Simply Sensational Blueberry Salad

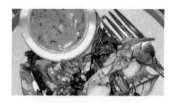

Prep Time: 15 Min.

Yield: 8 Servings

Ingredients	Amount	Measure	Have It	Need Qty
Fresh arugula	8	cups		
Blueberries	1 1/2	cups		
Pecans	3/4	cup		
Gorgonzola cheese	8	oz		
D'Anjou pears	2	pears		
Lemon	1	lemon		
Dijon mustard	1	tablespoon		
Olive oil	1/2	cup		
Champagne vinegar	3	tablespoons		

Instructions

1. Begin by prepping the pears. Peel and dice the pears and place them in a small mixing bowl. Squeeze a splash of fresh lemon over them to keep from browning.
2. In a blender, add the champagne vinegar, Dijon mustard, ½ the blueberries, and start the blender on low. Slowly drizzle in the olive oil through the pouring spout on the blender lid.
3. In a large bowl, place all the arugula, the pears, gorgonzola cheese, and pecans.
4. Pour in the dressing and toss all the ingredients together.
5. Top the salad with the remaining blueberries and serve.

Veggie Kabob

Prep Time: 45 Min.
Yield: 4 Servings

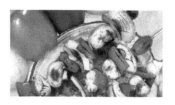

Ingredients	Amount	Measure	Have It	Need Qty
Fresh red peppers	2	peppers		
Fresh green peppers	2	peppers		
White onion	1	onion		
Mushrooms	1	pint		
Grape tomatoes	1	pint		
Olive oil	4	tablespoons		
Smoked paprika	1	tablespoons		
Salt & pepper		as desired		

Instructions

1. Prepare wooden skewers by placing them in a warm water bath in a container for 30 minutes to prevent burning.
2. Chop peppers into 1 inch pieces.
3. Chop mushrooms in half.
4. Chop the onion into 1 inch chunks.
5. Once the wooden skewers are thoroughly soaked, add vegetables to skewer alternating between red peppers, onion, grape tomatoes, mushroom, and green peppers. Add 2 layers per skewer.
6. Heat up the griddle on high heat. Once hot, reduce heat to medium high and brush griddle with olive oil. Brush each kabob with olive oil. Sprinkle salt, pepper, and smoky paprika and grill about 10-12 minutes or until vegetables are well grilled.

Balsamic Brussel Sprouts & Tomatoes

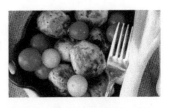

Prep Time: 30 Min.

Yield: 4 Servings

Ingredients	Amount	Measure	Have It	Need Qty
Balsamic vinegar	6	tablespoons		
Brussel sprouts	1	pound		
Cherry tomatoes	1	pint		
Shallots	2	shallots		
Kosher salt	1/2	teaspoon		
Onion powder	4	teaspoons		

Instructions

1. Bring 6 cups water to a boil in a stock pot with salt and onion powder. Add the cleaned Brussel sprouts. Boil for 8 min. (this will remove the bitterness)

2. In a sauté pan, add a splash of olive oil and shallots, cook for 2 minutes.

3. Drain the Brussel sprouts and add to the sauté pan.

4. Add balsamic vinegar and cook stirring occasionally every 2 minutes.

5. Cook for 10 minutes. Add the cherry tomatoes and cover for 5 additional minutes.

6. When the balsamic vinegar is thickened, serve and enjoy.

Health Conscious Deviled Eggs

Prep Time: 20 Min.
Yield: 4 Servings

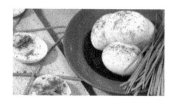

Ingredients	Amount	Measure	Have It	Need Qty
Organic eggs	6	eggs		
Greek yogurt	1/2	cup		
Dijon mustard	1	tablespoon		
Kosher salt	1	pinch		
Ground pepper		as desired		
Fresh chives	3	tablespoons		
Smoked paprika	1	tablespoons		
Onion powder	1/2	teaspoon		

Instructions

1. Place eggs in a pot of cold water. Turn on burner to medium heat.
2. Bring water to rolling boil and turn off the burner.
3. Place lid on pot and leave eggs in hot water for 15 minutes.
4. After 15 minutes, drain the water and add cold water.
5. Peel the eggs and rinse to ensure all shell is removed.
6. Slice all eggs in half.
7. Remove yolk and place in small mixing bowl.
8. Add Greek yogurt, Dijon mustard, kosher salt, and onion power to the yolks.
9. Fill each half egg white with a portion of the yolk mixture.
10. Top with fresh ground pepper, smoky paprika, and fresh chives.

Farm Fresh Vegetable Stew

Prep Time: 25 Min.
Yield: 8 Servings

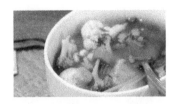

Ingredients	Amount	Measure	Have It	Need Qty
Olive oil	2	tablespoons		
White onion	1	onion		
Broccoli	3	bunches		
Caulliflower	1	head		
Celery	4	stalks		
Fresh garlic	4	cloves		
Mushrooms	1	pint		
Carrots	6	carrots		
Fresh parsley	2	bunches		
Chicken stock	16	oz		
Fresh corn	8	oz		
White wine	1	cup		

Instructions

1. In a large stock pot (Medium heat), add olive oil, diced onion, ½ tsp. salt.
2. Cook onion until opaque.
3. Add celery, carrots, garlic, mushrooms, and corn to pot and continue cooking for 6-8 min.
4. Once vegetables are cooked, add white wine. Allow vegetables to cook in white wine for 2 min.
5. Add chicken stock. Simmer on low for 20 min.
6. Add cauliflower and broccoli and cook for 10 additional minutes.
7. Top with fresh parsley and serve.

Dinners

Rosemary Chicken & Cauliflower Rice
Grapes & Chicken
Lemon Tilapia & Portobello
Ginger Soy Salmon
Rustic Lasagna
Angel Hair Pasta, Mushrooms & Shrimp
Spinach & Ricotta Ravioli
NM Red Chile Vegetarian Enchiladas
Hatch Green Chile Enchiladas

Rosemary & Chicken Cauliflower Rice

Prep Time: 20 Min.
Yield: 4 Servings

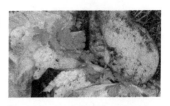

Ingredients	Amount	Measure	Have It	Need Qty
Chicken breasts	4	breasts		
Endive	20	leaves		
Caulliflower	1	head		
Fresh rosemary	2	bunches		
Fresh parsley	2	bunches		
Poultry seasoning	4	tablespoons		
Vegetable stock	3	cups		

Instructions

1. In a stock pot, bring the vegetable stock to a rolling boil.
2. Add the cauliflower and place the lid on the pot.
3. After 10 minutes, or until soft, remove from the liquid and place onto a plate with paper towel. Set aside.
4. In a mixing bowl, place the chicken and sprinkle the poultry seasoning, and 6 sprigs of rosemary. Cover with plastic wrap, marinade 20 minutes.
5. Cook the chicken on medium high heat until chicken is firm, or about 12-16 minutes. (the firmness of the palm of your hand is a good gauge, and the temperature should be 165 degrees at the thickest part of the chicken)
6. Using a food processor, pulse the cauliflower until it is the consistency of rice.
7. Plate the meal by placing cauliflower in endive cups. Place the chicken on the side, and top with fresh herbs.

Grapes & Chicken

Prep Time: 40 Min.
Yield: 4 Servings

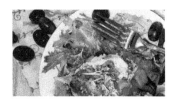

Ingredients	Amount	Measure	Have It	Need Qty
Chicken breast				
Red onion				
Shallots				
Fresh thyme				
Red grapes				
Fresh lemon				
White wine				
Poultry seasoning				
Olive oil				

Instructions

1. Marinade chicken ahead of time using lemon juice (from 1 lemon), 1 tbsp. olive oil, and poultry seasoning. Cover in plastic wrap and place in the refrigerator until cook time, but no less than 20 minutes.

2. In a cast iron skillet, on Medium high heat, place chicken breasts. Cook on the first side for 4 minutes. Turn the chicken and cook 3 additional minutes. Remove from the skillet and place on a plate and allow it to rest until time to place it back in the skillet.

3. In the same cast iron skillet, add olive oil, onion or *Shallots. Add ½ tsp. salt to sweat the onions. Cook for 3-5 minutes or until onions are soft.

4. Add grapes and thyme.

5. Add slices of fresh lemon and lemon zest.

6. Add the white wine to deglaze the pan, add chicken back to the skillet.

7. Cover and cook for 15 minutes.

8. Once finished, spoon the natural juices on top of finished chicken.

Lemon Tilapia & Portobello

Prep Time: 30 Min.
Yield: 6 Servings

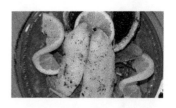

Ingredients	Amount	Measure	Have It	Need Qty
Tilapia	6	filets		
Portobello mushroom	6	mushrooms		
Fresh green beans	1	pound		
Lemon	2	lemons		
Salt & pepper	1/2	teaspoon (each)		
Olive oil	2	tablespoons		

Instructions

1. Wipe the mushrooms and brush them with extra virgin olive oil.

2. In a sauté pan on medium high, cook the mushrooms without the stem for 4 minutes on each side.

3. On a plate, lay out the tilapia and season simply with salt and pepper.

4. In a separate sauté pan, cook the tilapia for 2 minutes on each side on medium high. ONLY TURN THEM ONCE.

5. In a large stock pot, bring 6 cups of water to a boil. Add ½ cup of salt. Add the green beans for just 3 minutes.

6. Once the 3 minutes are up, remove the green beans and place them in a large bowl of ice water just for a minute.

7. Remove the green beans from the ice water and sauté them in a pan for just 2 minutes in a splash of olive oil.

8. Lay all on plate and top with fresh squeezed lemon and lemon slices.

Ginger Soy Salmon

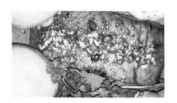

Prep Time: 20 Min.
Yield: 4 Servings

Ingredients	Amount	Measure	Have It	Need Qty
Fresh salmon	4	steaks		
Low sodium soy sauce	1/2	cup		
Fresh ginger	4	oz		
Sesame oil	4	tablespoons		
Sesame seeds	2	tablespoons		
Fresh lemon	1	lemon		
Pecans	1/3	cup		
Salt & pepper		as desired		

Instructions

1. Start by marinating the salmon 2 hours ahead of time. In a Pyrex bowl, place fresh salmon, ginger, soy sauce, sesame oil, sesame seeds, juice and zest of lemon. (cover with plastic wrap and keep in refrigerator for 2 hours)

2. Place the pecans in a Ziploc bag and using a rolling pin, crush them to pea size pieces. Put the pecans on a plate.

3. Once the salmon is ready to cook, place the fish on the pecans so the nuts stick to the fish.

4. Time to grill! On a griddle on medium to high heat, brush the grill with sesame oil. Place the salmon skin side up. Allow the salmon to cook 2 minutes then turn to the skin side down. Cook 2 additional minutes.

5. Squeeze fresh lemon on each piece and serve.

6. Add salt and pepper as desired.

Rustic Lasagna

Prep Time: 30 Min.
Yield: 4 Servings

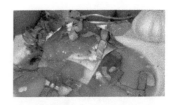

Ingredients	Amount	Measure	Have It	Need Qty
Lasagna noodles	4	each		
Fresh ricotta cheese	1 1/2	cup		
Fresh parmesan	6	oz		
Fresh romano	6	oz		
Fresh basil	2	bunches		
Olive oil	4	tablespoons		
Chicken stock	4	cups		
Crushed tomatoes	1	28oz can		
White onion	1	onion		
Fresh garlic	4	cloves		
Oregano	1	tablespoon		
Red pepper flakes	1/4	teaspoon		
Raw sugar	1	teaspoon		

Instructions

Marinara Sauce

1. In a medium sauce pan, heat up 2 tsp. olive oil, 2 minced garlic cloves, and 1 diced onion. Cook on medium heat for 5 minutes.
2. Add the crushed red tomatoes, ½ tbsp. salt and ½ tsp. raw sugar.
3. Add black pepper, crushed red pepper flakes, and oregano.
4. Cook an additional 10 minutes.

Lasagna

1. In a large stock pot, bring the chicken stock to a rolling boil on high heat. Add a splash of olive oil to prevent the noodles from sticking together.
2. In a separate bowl, mix the Ricotta, Parmesan, and Romano cheeses together.
3. Once the lasagna noodles are cooked (about 7 minutes) drain and lay them flat on a cutting board. Spoon the cheese mixture on one side of the noodle. Roll up the lasagna noodle and place 1 ladle full of marinara sauce on top. Roll up basil leaves and chop them. Sprinkle basil on top and bake covered for 20 minutes. Remove the foil and cook an additional 5 minutes.
4. Remove and place fresh basil on top, and Serve!

Angel Hair Pasta Mushrooms & Shrimp

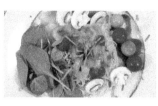

Prep Time: 35 Min.

Yield: 8 Servings

Ingredients	Amount	Measure	Have It	Need Qty
Angel hair pasta	8	oz		
Shrimp	1	pound		
Fresh basil	4	oz		
Fresh mushrooms	1	pint		
Cherry tomatoes	1	pint		
Chicken stock	6	cups		
Roma tomatoes	4	tomatoes		
Spinach	6	oz		
Fresh chives	4	oz		
Olive oil	6	tablespoons		
White onion	1	onion		
Parmesan cheese	6	oz		

Instructions

1. In a large stock pot, bring chicken stock to a rolling boil. Add 1 tbsp. olive oil and a 8-oz. package of angel hair. (Boil 5-6 minutes, until tender)
2. In a medium sauce pan, heat 2 tbsp. olive oil. Sauté 1 large diced onion.
3. Add halved cherry tomatoes and diced Roma tomatoes.
4. In a third sauté pan, sauté mushrooms, fresh basil and shrimp. Cook until the shrimp are pink.
5. Combine the mushroom mixture and tomatoes.
6. Add the cooked angel hair pasta and top with parmesan cheese, basil, and chives.

Spinach & Ricotta Ravioli

Prep Time: 1 Hr.
Yield: 4 Servings

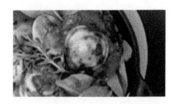

Ingredients	Amount	Measure	Have It	Need Qty
Gluten free all purpos flour				
Eggs				
Spinach				
Ricotta cheese				
Tomatoes				
Fresh parsley				
Oregano				
Fresh garlic				
White onion				

Instructions

Sauce

1. In a medium stock pot, sauté ½ diced onion in a splash of olive oil & ½ tsp. salt.
2. Once the onion is opaque, add garlic, minced. Cook on medium heat for 2 min.
3. Chop the tomatoes, and add them to the pot. Cook for 30 minutes on low heat.
4. Add oregano and keep on simmer.

Filling

1. In a medium sauté pan, sauté ½ an onion in olive oil, and half the spinach. Add 2 minced garlic cloves. Cook 8-10 minutes. Let it cool.
2. In a small mixing bowl, add cooked vegetable mixture and the ricotta cheese

Ravioli

1. In a stand mixer, add the flour and turn the mixer on low. Use the dough hook. Add a pinch of salt and the eggs. Mix oil well incorporated. (dough ball will form)
2. Roll out the dough if you don't have a pasta sheeter.
3. Using a circle cookie cutter (2 inch) cut our circles of dough. To each one add ½ tsp. of filling. Place a second pasta circle on top and crimp it with your fingers or use a fork.
4. In a pot of boiling water, cook the ravioli for 10 minutes.
5. Plate some ravioli and top with marinara sauce.
6. Add fresh parsley to the top!

NM Red Chile Vegetarian Enchiladas

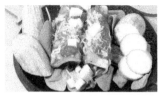

Prep Time: 45 Min.
Yield: 8 Servings

Ingredients	Amount	Measure	Have It	Need Qty
White corn tortillas	4	tortillas		
Fresh mushrooms	1	pint		
Mexican squash	2	squash		
Yellow squash	2	squash		
Fresh corn	2	ears		
Fresh spinach	8	oz		
Mild cheddar cheese	8	oz		
New Mexico red chiles	4	cups		
Vegetable stock	1	cup		
Fresh onion	1	cup		
Fresh garlic	4	cloves		
Oatmeal	1 1/2	cups		

Instructions

Chile Sauce

1. In a food processor, put 1 cup of oatmeal and grind to a powder. (set aside)
2. In a sauce pan, add 10 dried New Mexico red chile pods.
3. To that pan, add 2 cloves garlic and ½ chopped onion. Bring to a boil until chile pods have re-hydrated.
4. In a blender or food processor, blend the chile until liquefied.
5. In a separate large sauce pan, add the chile liquid, vegetable stock, and oatmeal.
6. Bring to a rolling boil until thickened.
7. Add salt to taste.

Filling

1. On a grill, char 2 ears of corn on the cob (set aside to cool).
2. In a medium sauté pan, heat up 1 tsp. olive oil., add diced onion, mushrooms, Mexican & yellow squash, onion, and garlic, sauté until the vegetables are soft.
3. Remove the corn from the cob and add to the mixture.
4. Add the spinach to the pan and allow to wilt. Set aside.

Enchilada

1. Warm the corn tortillas on a hot plate until soft.
2. Place 2 tbsp. of filling in each tortilla and roll.
3. Put 1 ladle of Chile sauce on top. Sprinkle 1 Oz. of cheese and serve

Hatch Green Chili Enchiladas

Prep Time: 1 Hr.

Yield: 4 Servings

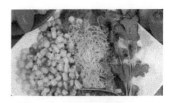

Ingredients	Amount	Measure	Have It	Need Qty
White corn tortillas	4	tortillas		
Fresh mushrooms	1	pint		
Mexican squash	4	squash		
Sharp cheddar cheese	4	oz		
Fresh onion	1	onion		
Fresh jalapeño	1	small		
Hatch chiles	8	oz		
Chicken stock	2	cups		
Beef stock	2	cups		
Oatmeal	1	cup		
White onion	1	large onion		
Fresh garlic	4	cloves		
Fresh cilantro	3	tablespoons		

Instructions

Chile Sauce

1. In a food processor, put 1 cup of oatmeal and grind to a powder (set aside).
2. Dice 1 large onion and sauté in 1 tbsp. olive oil.
3. Add roasted, peeled and chopped Hatch green chile.
4. Add fresh garlic.
5. Add the ground oatmeal.
6. Add both the chicken and beef stock.
7. Bring to a rolling boil until thickened. Add salt to taste and cilantro if desired.

Filling

1. In a medium sauté pan, heat 1 tsp. olive oil, diced onion, mushrooms, and Mexican squash.
2. Slice the jalapeno in half and remove the rib and seeds.
3. Chop finely and add to the mixture. Cook until vegetables are soft.

Enchilada

1. Warm the corn tortillas on a hot plate until soft.
2. Place 2 tbsp. of filling in each tortilla and roll.
3. Put 1 ladle of Chile sauce on top. Sprinkle 1 Oz. of cheese and serve

Desserts

Fresh Cinnamon Apple Pie
Fresh Blueberry Pie (Slim Version)
Pumpkin Pie on the Lighter Side

Fresh Cinnamon Apple Pie

Prep Time: 45 Min.
Yield: 8 Servings

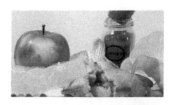

Ingredients	Amount	Measure	Have It	Need Qty
Almond flour	2	cups		
Coconut oil	2	tablespoons		
Egg	1	egg		
Salt	1/4	teaspoon		
Fresh sliced fuji apples	4	cups		
Coconut sugar	1/2	cup		
Fresh lemon	1	juice and zest		
Cinnamon	1/4	tablespoon		
Salt	1/4	teaspoon		

Instructions

Pie Crust
1. In a mixing bowl, add almond flour, salt, coconut oil, and egg.
2. Mix until well incorporated.
3. Place half the dough in a pie plate and hand form the dough to the plate at about 1/8-inch thickness.
4. Save the other half of the dough for the top layer of crust.

Filling
5. In a mixing bowl, add apple slices, lemon, cinnamon, coconut sugar and salt.
6. Combine well.
7. Pour filling into prepared pie shell.
8. Place rolled out top layer of crust on pie.
9. For best results, beat 1 egg white and brush the top of the pie before baking.
10. Sprinkle ½ tsp. coconut sugar on top.
11. Bake for 14-16 minutes at 340 degrees or until golden brown.

Fresh Blueberry Pie
Slim Version

Prep Time: 45 Min.
Yield: 8 Servings

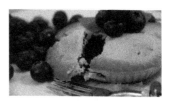

Ingredients	Amount	Measure	Have It	Need Qty
Almond flour	2	cups		
Coconut oil	2	tablespoons		
Egg	1	egg		
Salt	1/4	teaspoon		
Fresh blueberries	5	cups		
Maple syrup	1/3	cup		
Fresh lemon	1	juice and zest		
Cinnamon	1/4	tablespoon		
Salt	1/4	teaspoon		

Instructions

Pie Crust

1. In a mixing bowl, add almond flour, salt, coconut oil, and egg.
2. Mix until well incorporated.
3. Place half the dough in a pie plate and hand form the dough to the plate at about 1/8-inch thickness.
4. Save the other half of the dough for the top layer of crust.

Filling

5. In a mixing bowl, add fresh blueberries, maple syrup, lemon juice and zest, cinnamon, and salt.
6. With a wooden spoon, mix all ingredients well.
7. Pour into pie shell.
8. Place rolled out top layer of crust on pie.
9. For best results, beat 1 egg white and brush the top of the pie before baking.
10. Bake for 14-16 minutes at 360 degrees or until golden brown.
11. Serve.

Pumpkin Pie on the Lighter side

Prep Time: 45 Min.
Yield: 8 Servings

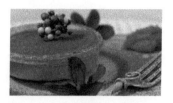

Ingredients	Amount	Measure	Have It	Need Qty
Almond flour	1 1/2	cups		
Salt	1	pinch		
Coconut sugar	1/3	cup		
Butter	1/2	cup		
Iced water	3/4	tablespoons		
Pumpkin puree	1	16oz can		
Full fat cocounut mil	1	13oz can		
Rolled oats	1/4	cup		
Coconut sugar	1/3	cup		
Cinnamon	2	teaspoons		
Pumpkin pie spice	1	teaspoon		
Vanilla extract	2	teaspoons		
Salt	1/2	teaspoon		

Instructions

Pie Crust

1. In a food processor, add almond flour, salt, coconut sugar, and COLD butter.
2. Pulse until the butter is incorporated to the size of small peas.
3. Add 1 tbsp. ICE COLD water until a ball forms.
4. Remove the dough and wrap in plastic wrap.
5. Place dough in refrigerator for 30 minutes.
6. After 30 minutes, remove dough and roll out on a floured surface.
7. Place dough in a pie plate and form it to the pan.
8. Bake the crust at 320 degrees for 6-8 minutes until LIGHTLY brown. It will cook more after the filling is added.

Filling

1. In a mixing bowl, add the pumpkin puree, coconut milk, coconut sugar, cinnamon, pumpkin pie spice, salt, and vanilla.
2. In a food processor, process the ¼ cup rolled oats for 1 minute until a powder.
3. Add the oatmeal to the pumpkin mixture (filling will thicken during baking).
4. Pour mixture into the cooked pie shell and bake for 12-15 minutes at 360 degrees.Once your pie is baked, it will look underbred. Place in refrigerator for 4 hours. Slice and enjoy

9

Portion Your Plate

I've mentioned the importance of "portion control," which is understanding how much a serving size of food is and how many calories is contained in a single serving of food. In order for you to be successful in your weight-loss endeavor, portion control will be absolutely crucial to your victory.

In 1970, Americans ate an average of 2,000 calories per day. Fast forward to 2010, the latest year we have statistics, and we learn that Americans upped that number to more than 2,600 calories per day. To give a few examples, a bagel in the 1970s was about three inches in diameter and had 140 calories. Today, bagels have doubled in size and more than doubled in calories to 350 calories.

Soda is another prime example of how portion sizes have increased over the years. In the 1970s, the average soda serving was 6.5 ounces with 65 calories. Today, you can buy cans of soda with serving sizes of 20 ounces, which have 250 calories. I shake my head as I remember how at McDonald's we were trained to ask customers if they wanted to "supersize" their meals with bigger sodas and more fries. Although that's no longer the case today, supersizing meals added a lot of calories.

Too many calories, I'm afraid. The USDA recommends that the average moderately active male human being should consume 2,600 calories per day and women should consume 2,000 calories per day, but the average American exceeds those numbers by several hundred calories a day.

There was no need to count calories back in ancient times, when cavemen had to burn calories to catch their food. Many experts today tell us that we should eat a "stone age" or "paleo" diet, which means eating all the lean meat and all the seafood you want as well as fruits, berries, and vegetables that don't contain starch.

We're no longer "hunters and gatherers" who depend on hunting animals, and we're not even an agricultural society like we were 120 years ago in 1900 when 38 percent of the work force was involved in farming. Industrial growth has transformed the way we live and work, and the mechanization of the way we produce food has changed farming forever.

Now, only 2 percent of Americans are involved in agricultural . . . and the rest of us sit in cubicles or work in service industry jobs like I do in the restaurant world. What I'm trying to say is that we essentially don't do any physical work, which means we're burning barely any calories during the day.

The lack of movement also means we are also storing fat cells. Fat cells are nothing more than power for our bodies. Think of them as battery power. Going back to ancient times, the cavemen also had fat cells, but they walked so much in a search for food that they didn't store fat cells like we do today.

These days, I'm afraid that we have evolved and "perfected" the fat cell, which seems to multiply and multiply. My overall concern with the current human diet is that as we get closer to 2020, we will work even less to eat. It is difficult to imagine what the next generation will face.

Going back to the USDA recommendations is important. The self-reported intake of calories is close to 2,600 calories for men and 2,000 calories for women, but that's "self-reporting." The figure has to be considerably higher since so many people are overweight. And it's easy to eat too many calories, especially if your diet is built around processed food and eating at fast food restaurants.

The antidote to overeating—oops, I mean consuming too many calories—is to practice portion control.

Listen, we all love food. Many people go on holiday and plan their time around food and eating, from cruise ships to fortnights in the Tuscany region of Italy, where pasta and pizza reign. But if you're going to lose weight and *keep* it off, you need to be thinking about consuming 1,000 calories a day.

A thousand calories a day. Aren't I going to starve?

Based upon my personal experience, I would say no. I've found it quite possible to live a full life on 1,000 calories and function properly. One thousand calories a day can sustain you.

This means you will have to count calories and "portion" them out throughout the day. That's what I mean by "portion control." A 1,000-calorie diet may not work for everyone, but it's important you know how much you're eating throughout the day and night. If you happen to participate in strenuous exercise, you can consume a few more calories, but make sure they are high protein foods. Eliminate sugary drinks completely.

A typical 1,000-calorie per day diet includes three servings of grains, two servings of protein, two servings of fruit, five servings of veggies, two servings of milk, and 2 teaspoons of vegetable oil. Some great grain choices would include one slice of whole grain bread or about 3 to 4 tablespoons of dried oats. The fruit portion size should be about 1 cup of fruit, or a medium-size apple or orange. The serving size of vegetables should be 1 cup of raw veggies or 1/2 cup of cooked veggies.

To stay on track with a 1,000-calorie diet, it's essential that you not waste your calories on ingredients such as mayonnaise or sauces. Stay hydrated with water, which is beneficial to our overall health. Drinking soda is not an option and shouldn't even be considered as a "treat" or as a "cheat day" item.

Sorry, ladies, but men can consume more calories because men burn calories faster than women. That said, it's important that you space out your meals so that your body doesn't go into starvation mode, which can be harmful to your health. Once your body goes into starvation mode, it thinks that you will no longer feed it, so it holds all the fat cells in reserve (remember the analogy of the battery) just in case your body needs them in the future.

One way I prevent my body from going into starvation mode is by making sure I eat a very small breakfast or a protein drink within thirty minutes of waking up to kick-start my metabolism. This is the most important thing that we as humans can do for our health. The rest of the day, I eat small meals regularly. I find that five or six small meals a day keeps me going.

You should also use small plates when enjoying a meal—since it will look like you have more food than you think. I recommend that your plates be no larger than six inches in diameter. You might want to pack up your large plates and put them in your attic.

Make meal time enjoyable. Eat healthy foods that matter—lean meat, veggies, and fruit. These foods provide your body with the fuel you need. Control the portions at each meal by taking only one serving from each food group.

The best way to not drink calories is to drink water, which is calorie-free since it doesn't contain any fats, carbohydrates, or proteins. Use small glasses that can hold a maximum of 8 ounces of water.

When eating out, ask for a take-out container before you begin your meal. Put aside at least half the meal and eat the other half at another meal-time sitting. As a bariatric survivor, I still do not combine food and drinks. This is a habit that we should all practice. Allow your body to keep the nutrients from your foods without the disruption of liquids pushing it through your body too quickly.

Eat to live a healthy life, instead of living to eat. And always remember to portion your plate!

ACKNOWLEDGEMENTS

No person in this life ever walks alone—or should walk alone. Over the course of my life, I've been fortunate to have many people walking alongside me. Most significant are my immediate family members: my father, Manuel, my mother, Gloria, and my siblings, Anthony and Jeannette. They have always been there for me, offering support and guidance through the ups and downs of my journey. I am extremely grateful to you all.

I also want to publicly thank my mother, who has always been my strongest supporter and has showed me what it is to love unconditionally. Better yet, she is and always has been my biggest fan. So, Mom, I'm very thankful God chose you to be my mother. I love you more than words can express!

About the Author

Jacob Bustos is a chef, cooking coach, and food enthusiast who has been in the food business for twenty-four years. Jacob, who has always been passionate about hospitality, beat his battle with morbid obesity and has set out to make a positive impact on people. He will tell you that as long as you know him, he will

never let you go hungry. This is true to his mission that food is love, family, and fellowship. He will also be the first to tell you how important healthy food choices are.

Jacob began his career in the fast food business and earned various awards for great customer service. He left the fast food business in 2002 and currently works in upper management for a number of fast-causal Panera Bread restaurants in the Southern California area.

Jacob underwent a life-saving bariatric procedure in 2012 that began his 160-pound weight loss journey. He also underwent a traumatic skin removal surgery in 2015 that nearly ended his life. During this traumatic event, he had a very private and personal experience with his Maker that affirmed his mission on earth to feed people with much healthier options.

Jacob has been in demand for speaking engagements and has produced videos to teach and coach better eating habits. His ability to take a regular food dish and create a healthier version have been in high demand. For more information on Jacob and his company, Portion Your Plate LLC, please visit www.JacobBustos.com or www.PortionYourPlate.com.

Jacob resides in Valencia, California, just north of Los Angeles.

INVITE JACOB BUSTOS

to Speak Today

Jacob Bustos is a dynamic speaker with a passion to inspire all generations about healthy eating and about weight loss surgery. He has spoken all over the United States about his journey to weight loss and his personal health. Jacob has a passion to help the next generation live a full, healthy, and happy life.

If you, your community group, college or university, or high school would be interested in having Jacob speak, please contact his agents, George Baker and Carter Dandridge, at ASAP Talent Agency via e-mail at gb@asap101.com and carter@asap101.com, respectively, or visit the agency's website at www.asaptalentagency.com.

Resource List

The below resources are provided for more detailed health and statistical information on diseases and conditions such as obesity, diabetes and heart disease, in addition to helpful research sites on bariatric procedures.

American Heart Association
http://www.heart.org/HEARTORG/
American Liver Foundation - http://www.liverfoundation.org/abouttheliver/info/progression/
American Society for Metabolic and Bariatric Surgery
https://asmbs.org
Centers for Disease Control and Prevention
https://www.cdc.gov
Diabetes Research Institute Foundation
https://www.diabetesresearch.org
Johns Hopkins Medicine
http://www.hopkinsmedicine.org
Mayo Clinic
http://www.mayoclinic.org
National Institutes of Health
https://www.nih.gov/health-information

9 781642 793376